Gerontological Nurse

Certification Review

Alison E. Kris, PhD, RN, is an associate professor of nursing at Fairfield University where she has taught numerous courses at the undergraduate and graduate levels, including research methods, biostatistics, geriatrics, pathophysiology, and pharmacology. She has participated in interdisciplinary research through Fairfield University's Integrative Nursing and Health Studies Initiative, where she directed a team of undergraduate research assistants and supervised doctoral-level coursework and undergraduate theses. She has extensive research and clinical experience and has published numerous scholarly articles and book chapters. She received her bachelor of science in nursing from the University of Pennsylvania; her PhD from the University of California, San Francisco; and she was awarded a postdoctoral fellowship from the John A. Hartford Foundation, which she completed at the University of California, San Francisco.

Gerontological Nurse

Certification Review

Second Edition

Alison E. Kris, PhD, RN

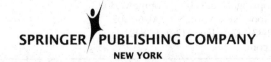

SPRINGER PUBLISHING COMPANY
NEW YORK

Springer Publishing Company, LLC
11 West 42nd Street
New York, NY 10036
www.springerpub.com

Acquisitions Editor: Elizabeth Nieginski
Composition: diacriTech

ISBN: 978-0-8261-3017-4
e-book ISBN: 978-0-8261-3018-1

15 16 17 18/ 5 4 3 2 1

The author and the publisher of this Work have made every effort to use sources believed to be reliable to provide information that is accurate and compatible with the standards generally accepted at the time of publication. Because medical science is continually advancing, our knowledge base continues to expand. Therefore, as new information becomes available, changes in procedures become necessary. We recommend that the reader always consult current research and specific institutional policies before performing any clinical procedure. The author and publisher shall not be liable for any special, consequential, or exemplary damages resulting, in whole or in part, from the readers' use of, or reliance on, the information contained in this book. The publisher has no responsibility for the persistence or accuracy of URLs for external or third-party Internet websites referred to in this publication and does not guarantee that any content on such websites is, or will remain, accurate or appropriate.

Library of Congress Cataloging-in-Publication Data
Kris, Alison E., author.
Gerontological nurse certification review / Alison E. Kris. — Second edition.
    p. ; cm.
 Preceded by: Gerontological nurse certification review / Meredith Wallace, Sheila Grossman. c2008.
 Includes bibliographical references and index.
  ISBN 978-0-8261-3017-4 — ISBN 978-0-8261-3018-1 (e-book)
 I. Kazer, Meredith Wallace Gerontological nurse certification review. Preceded by (work): II. Title.
[DNLM: 1. Geriatric Nursing — Examination Questions. 2. Geriatric Assessment — Examination Questions.
WY 18.2]
RC954
618.97'0231 — dc23

                 2015000193

Printed in the United States of America by Bradford & Bigel

Contents

Foreword

For several decades, policy experts and health care professionals have made projections regarding the coming baby boomer bubble of an aging American population, detailing dramatic changes in the size and composition of this American population and the challenges this will create for all health care professionals. Those projections have come to fruition, creating an urgent need for health care professionals, and nurses in particular, to have a strong base of knowledge and skills in care of older adults. Demographic realities will create an increase of adults older than the age of 65 in the very near term, adding to the increasing number of individuals in this country who are termed the "oldest old."

The aging of America has created a dynamic and changing perspective on aging. Older adults are living longer while maintaining full employment, and active social and community lives. However, this longevity is accompanied by a concurrent increase in chronic illnesses treated with sophisticated technological and pharmacological interventions. This enormously complex array of treatments creates the need for a health professional workforce that is prepared to meet the unique physiological and psychosocial needs of older adults. The unique skill sets that are required to provide safe, high-quality, and effective care to older adults are not intuitively acquired, but rather come only from a focused approach to developing new views and knowledge to shape and define how care is delivered to the older adult.

Unfortunately, despite the growth in the population of older adults, the nursing profession has not seen a concomitant increase in the proportion of the nursing workforce with a specialization in geriatrics. Increasingly, however, nurses and other professionals are seeking the specific skill sets necessary to deliver high-quality care to older adults. Much of the enhanced focus on geriatrics comes as a result of the important and substantial support that has been made available to the nursing profession by the John A. Hartford Foundation. Through this support, an enhanced focus on both geriatric practice and research has blossomed in the profession, and nursing professionals have increasingly sought the specific knowledge and skills necessary to meet this challenge. As nurses seek this knowledge, they also seek professional validation as a specialized geriatric clinician represented by certification by a national body. Certification is an external validation of competence to meet specific and important needs and is the hallmark of excellence in nursing practice.

This fully updated publication is an important addition to the resources available for nurses who seek certification as geriatric clinicians. This resource, designed for the generalist baccalaureate-educated nursing clinician who desires validation through expert knowledge and skills for the care of the older adult, also recognizes the reality of practice. Generalist practice is almost uniformly geriatric practice. The preponderance of older adults in today's acute care facilities, long-term care settings, and communities should create awareness among all nursing professionals that the knowledge and skills assessed through geriatric certification are a basic foundation for safe practice today.

In this book, the tools and clear presentation of information related to the actual testing process provide the learner with a framework for confidence as he or she prepares for the exam. More important, however, is the elaborate presentation of the certification content and the attention to the important physical and psychosocial elements of the human aging process.

The American Nurses Association (ANA) Scope and Standards of Practice Statement expresses clearly the central role nurses play in protecting and assuring that safe and effective care is delivered. This statement notes: "Today, as in the past, nursing remains pivotal in improving the health status of the public and ensuring safe, effective, quality care" (ANA, 2010). This mandate for nursing to engage in safe, effective, high-quality care for older adults cannot be met without a strong base of knowledge regarding the unique needs of this population. As nurses strive to engage in this level of practice, certification will validate the commitment to providing the best care possible. This book enables nursing professionals to acquire certification as a geriatric specialist and provides them with the ability to achieve this important and professionally responsible goal. Data from the Census Bureau tell us that there are currently approximately 39 million Americans age 65 and older, up from 25.5 million just 30 years ago. This population explosion is unprecedented in history, and the resulting demographic shift is causing profound social and economic changes.

Geraldine Bednash, PhD, RN, FAAN
Executive Director
American Association of Colleges of Nursing Washington, DC

REFERENCE

American Nurses Association. (2010). *Scope and standards of nursing practice* (2nd ed. Silver Springs, MD: ANA. http://www.nursesbooks.org/ebooks/download/ NursingScopeStandards.pdf

Preface

The *Gerontological Nurse Certification Review, Second Edition*, has been written as a reference and certification test review guide for RNs preparing for gerontological certification. It is also a useful text for students who are studying gerontology, teachers preparing gerontology classes, and RNs working with older adults. The book presents information about preparing for the certification exam, a comprehensive compilation of content specific to gerontology, and a test bank of questions specifically developed for the RN preparing for certification in gerontology.

Chapters 1 and 2 provide necessary step-by-step information for the certification candidate to prepare for and take the test. The remaining chapters, 3 through 13, are organized according to the various topics of the blueprint of the Gerontological Nurse Certification Exam for baccalaureate and associate degree nurses. Chapter 3 focuses on topics specific to the aging population, such as demographics, myths about aging, theories of aging and nursing, communication skills geared for the older adult, teaching–learning principles that work well with older adults, and the history of gerontological nursing. Chapter 4 describes the changes that go with normal aging and addresses questions referring to taking a history of and performing a physical exam on older adults. Chapter 5 identifies the health-promotion needs of elders, such as nutrition, exercise, primary and secondary prevention strategies, and alternative and complementary health care practices used with older adults. Chapter 6 describes the environment, including safety and security, relocation, transportation, the importance of space, community-based resources, and residential facilities. Spirituality and dying are discussed in Chapter 7 with special attention to advance directives, hospice and palliative care, and the grieving process. Chapter 8 describes the acute and chronic physical illnesses most frequently experienced by older adults. Chapter 9 discusses the cognitive and psychological disorders experienced by elders, including dementia, delirium, and depression. Common medications used by older adults, as well as discussions about polypharmacy, issues related to pharmacokinetics and pharmacodynamics, noncompliance, and adverse drug effects are covered in Chapter 10. Special topics such as pain, sexuality, and elder neglect and abuse are discussed in Chapter 11. Descriptions of health policy issues and organizations that advocate for older adults are covered in Chapter 12. Chapter 13 discusses the scope and standards of geriatric nursing practice relating to leadership and management, research, ethical and legal issues, and professional competency.

Finally, the Posttest contains 500 test questions, and it is followed by the correct answers with corresponding rationales covering the various content areas. Readers can choose to take the comprehensive integrated test under simulated timed conditions or they can select parts of the Posttest to take at different times, scheduled for the convenience of the individual.

The importance of practicing psychomotor skills, communicating with others, and increasing experience with various competencies such as leading, delegating, organizing, and assessing is clearly important to clinical success. Similarly, the practice of reading scenario questions and answering them is considered very important in achieving success on an exam. Moreover, with the increasing elder population, CCNE certification is essential to the availability of a nursing workforce educated in assessing and meeting the needs of older adults. The author hopes that all nurses who complete this preparation book will gain valuable knowledge, validate their competency on the certification test, and improve their ability to deliver high-quality care to older adults.

Alison E. Kris

1

Information for Taking the

Certification Exam

The *Gerontological Nurse Certification Review* prepares RNs to take the American Nurses Credentialing Center (ANCC) Gerontological Nursing Board Certification Examination. Candidates who successfully pass the exam will become board-certified RNs, and will receive the credential RN-BC. By obtaining gerontological certification, nurses gain power similar to board-certified physicians and advanced practice nurses. There is an incentive to become certified in one's area of expertise. Most institutions will apply certification toward promotion to the next staff level. Some institutions give a bonus or a differential pay raise for certification. If you are affiliated with a Magnet hospital that supports certification for professional development, you will be further recognized. Most important, certification is an excellent way to be recognized for expertise in a specialty area. It is highly likely your institution will reimburse you for the fee required to obtain certification status.

The purpose of this chapter is to explain:

- The ANCC testing format
- The application and scheduling of the test date for certification in gerontology
- General hints to improve your preparation for the exam

CERTIFICATION EXAM FORMAT

The ANCC offers a computer-based test in multiple-choice format with the option of choosing one of four possible answers. The test contains 150 questions and covers content knowledge and application of professional nursing regarding gerontology at an entry-level competency. The exam is developed from role-delineation studies that measure the necessary knowledge and skills needed for competent practice in a specialty area, such as gerontology (American Nurses Credentialing Center [ANCC], 2014). The purpose of the exam is to determine whether nurses are competent to assess the strengths of older adults in order to facilitate their highest quality of life and, when appropriate, a "good death." The ANCC updates the RN gerontology certification exam on a regular basis. A 75-question Practice Certification Examination with answers can be accessed at www.anfonline.org/ANF/geroexam.pdf. Completing the practice exam and reviewing your answers is strongly recommended.

Table 1.1 lists the 10 exam topic areas, the percentage of the test that correlates with each content, and the corresponding number of questions that are asked about each area.

DETAILED TEST CONTENT OUTLINE

This book is organized chapter by chapter according to the ANCC RN Gerontology Test Content Outline, which can be seen in detail at www .nursecredentialing.org/GeroNurse-TCO2015.

Total Number of Questions

There are 175 questions on the test, but 25 of them are pilot questions and do not count toward one's score. There is no way to determine which of the 175 questions count for your test, so it is best to consider each question as carefully as you can. This is the standard approach for validating new questions and ensuring that they are reliable.

TABLE 1.1 American Nurses Credentialing Center (ANCC) Domains of Practice

TOPIC AREA	PERCENTAGE OF THE EXAM	NUMBER OF QUESTIONS
Assessment	17.33	26
Plan of Care	23.33	35
Person-Centered Care	28.67	43
Professional Practice	14	21
Health Promotion	16.67	25

Adapted from the ANCC (2013).

Total Time

The time allowed to take the test is 3.5 hours. If desired, test takers can take a 20-minute practice exam to become oriented with the computer system. This is highly recommended for all test takers. This tutorial can be reviewed at the ANCC website, www.anfonline.org/ANF/geroexam.pdf. Most people complete the exam in about 2.5 hours, but ANCC allows 3.5 hours to take the exam.

ELIGIBILITY TO TAKE THE EXAM

To take the certification exam, you must provide payment (see the ANCC website for details about the cost), a copy of your current unrestricted RN license, documentation that you have practiced full time as an RN the equivalent of 2 years, have had a minimum of 2,000 hours of clinical practice in gerontology in the past 3 years, and the completed application. You must also provide documentation of 30 continuing-education hours in the gerontology specialty that you have acquired in the past 3 years. In case you are ever audited, it is recommended that you maintain a file of your continuing-education certificates. The application will request that you include a description of the continuing-education course and how it is relevant to your geriatric practice if the course title does not reflect gerontology clearly.

A *General Testing and Renewal Handbook* with testing information and an application can be accessed at www.nursecredentialing.org/GeroNursing-Application (ANCC, 2014). You can type directly onto the application and print it. The address to send the application is American Nurses Credentialing Center, PO Box 791333, Baltimore, MD, 21279-1333.

If you have any questions regarding the application, you can send an e-mail to certification@ana.org or call 1-800-284-2378 for further clarification and additional information.

SCHEDULING THE TEST

The test is administered by Thomson Prometric Computer Testing Centers. To choose a location, first set up a date and time to take the computerized test on Prometric's website (www.prometric.com/ANCC). An authorization to test (ATT) will be mailed to you from the testing center. After you receive the ATT, call 1-800-350-7076 or visit www.2test.com and make an appointment during the 90-day eligibility period stated on your ATT form.

Testing centers are located in every state and some locations in Canada, Puerto Rico, and Guam. You can schedule, reschedule, or cancel your appointment at the Prometric website. Hours for testing are generally 8 a.m. to 5 p.m., and the testing center is open Monday through Friday. It is recommended that you schedule your test appointment as soon as you get your ATT to guarantee the best opportunity of getting your desired day and time. If you decide to switch the date, time, or test-site location, you need to follow the directions in the ANCC *General Testing and Renewal Handbook* located at www.nursecredentialing.org/cert/PDFs/ExamHandbook.pdf.

WHAT TO BRING ON THE DAY OF THE EXAM

You need to bring your ATT form and two forms of identification that match the name on your ATT form. One form of ID must have your photo, and both forms must have your signature. One form must be your passport, a photo driver's license, or a photo government-issued ID card. You will not be admitted without the necessary forms of identification. You cannot take any personal items into the testing room. You will be provided with scratch paper and a pencil only. You will be given a locker to store your valuables, such as car keys and wallet.

TIME OF ARRIVAL

Test takers *must* arrive 15 minutes earlier than the scheduled test time. Failure to arrive early will cost you your appointment and require you to reapply.

DURING THE EXAM

There are no refreshment breaks. You can take a restroom break according to the instructions given at the testing center, but this time will be subtracted from your total time of 3.5 hours. You cannot ask any questions during the exam. When you complete the test, you cannot take the scratch paper from the testing room.

RECEIVING TEST RESULTS

You will be provided with your results before you leave the test center. The results of the exam are pass or fail. Those who fail the exam will receive a diagnostic explanation for each of the content areas.

RECEIVING CERTIFICATE AND PIN

Those who pass the exam receive a certificate, pin, and identification card that acknowledges ANCC certification within approximately 8 weeks. This certification is valid for 5 years. Information regarding recertification is available at www.nursecredentialing.org.

HINTS FOR TAKING THE CERTIFICATION EXAM

■ There is no penalty for guessing, so it is recommended that test takers answer every question. You may skip questions and come back to them later.

■ The test covers general and frequently seen gerontological problems, not rare and exotic diseases.

- Be familiar with the common drugs used by older adults.
- Know the frequently occurring adverse drug events for older adults and be able to apply the Modified Beers Criteria.
- You should know the normal laboratory results for the diseases that older adults commonly experience.

References that are recommended by the ANCC regarding gerontology are available at www.nursecredentialing.org or by calling 1-800-284-2378.

REFERENCES

American Nurses Credentialing Center. (2013, September 26). *ANCC gerontology certification exam content outline.* Retrieved from http://www.nursecredentialing .org/cert/TCOs/09Gero_TCO.html

American Nurses Credentialing Center. (2013). *2013 general testing and renewal handbook.* Retrieved from http://www.nursecredentialing.org/cert/PDFs/examhand book.pdf

American Nurses Credentialing Center. (2014). *2013 gerontological nursing role delineation study: National survey results.* Retrieved from http://www.nursecredentialing .org/Certification/NurseSpecialties/Gerontological/RELATED-LINKS/ GeroNursing-2013RDS.pdf

2

Question Dissection and Analysis

PREPARATION STRATEGIES

Preparing for a standardized exam can cause some anxiety and fear. It is necessary to remember that you are an experienced RN who has practiced full time as a registered nurse for the equivalent of 2 years or you have a minimum of 2,000 hours of clinical practice in gerontology in the past 3 years. Either way, you have some excellent expertise that you can draw on while preparing for this examination. You also have experience using the nursing process in many situations with older adults, so you already are experienced in

- Assessing situations and outcomes
- Analyzing situations and prioritizing
- Planning
- Implementing the plan of care
- Evaluating patient outcomes

Everything that you do in your mind when using the nursing process in your clinical practice, you will continue to do as you reason through the test questions.

A question may be designed to evaluate your assessment expertise or how you would prioritize and schedule care, a question may ask you to plan for a specific patient outcome given the data presented in the question, or you may be asked to choose the best way of caring for a condition. Some questions will depict a patient situation that needs evaluation. For all the questions, you will be critically thinking through the scenario using the nursing process. Your thought processes will mirror what you would have done in similar situations if you were at your work setting. Table 2.1 outlines the similarity of the thought processes that occur when taking the exam and being in practice.

TABLE 2.1 Performance in Clinical Practice Mirrors Thought Processes for Taking the Gerontological Nurse Certification Exam

CLINICAL PRACTICE	ANALYZING TEST QUESTION
Assess the patient with a comprehensive review of symptoms during admission or episodically.	Take the data that are significant for patient assessment from the question stem and match them with the point of the question.
Analyze all of the data you collected in assessment and use it to plan the patient's care.	Take the significant clues from the question stem and prioritize all of the information so that you can make the most appropriate plan.
Plan the care necessary to meet the patient's needs. Remember to make priorities.	Review the stem of the question and choose the information that tells you the patient's diagnosis, current status, and whether there is a priority situation that needs immediate attention. Analyze this together and select from the possible answers the plan that best fits the patient's needs.
Implement the plan with a possible need for rescheduling some actions given the patient's needs.	Take the significant clues in the stem of the question that indicate what the patient needs now and in the future. Analyze all of the information and choose the sequence of actions that you would take if this was your patient in practice.
Evaluate the patient's outcomes with respect to the appropriate plan that was implemented.	Review the stem of the question and brainstorm about what you would be evaluating given the diagnosis and patient status. Choose the answer based on the standards of care and evidence-based practice you follow in clinical practice.

REVIEW CONTENT OF FREQUENT CONDITIONS EXPERIENCED BY OLDER ADULTS

Some of the most significant content information necessary to competently care for older adults reflects assessing, analyzing, planning, implementing, and evaluating patient outcomes of conditions that older adults most frequently experience. These conditions are denoted as *red flag* problems. Older adult, red-flag problems are discussed in more detail in Chapter 8, "Acute and Chronic Physical Illnesses." You should review these areas carefully if you feel you do not have a competent level of knowledge regarding these conditions:

■ Heart failure

■ Hypertension

■ Hypotension

■ Coronary artery disease

■ Myocardial infarction

■ Peripheral vascular disease

■ Pneumonia

- Emphysema
- Constipation
- Diarrhea
- Gastroesophageal reflux disease
- Peptic ulcer disease
- Diverticulosis
- Benign prostatic hypertrophy
- Urinary incontinence
- Anemia
- Osteoporosis
- Osteoarthritis
- Hip fractures
- Diabetes mellitus
- Thyroid disease
- Common causes of confusion, including depression, delirium, and dementia
- Cerebrovascular accident
- Parkinson's disease

STRATEGIES FOR ANALYZING THE QUESTIONS

It is important to be familiar with the two parts of a question. The sentence or phrase that follows the question number is called the stem. Following the stem there are three incorrect answers called distracters as well as one correct answer. Many successful test takers cover the answers with a piece of paper or their hand and read the stem of the question without looking at the possible answer choices. After reading the stem, the test taker reflects on the question stem and thinks about what the answer might be. After reviewing the answer choices, the test taker can then choose the response most similar to what came to mind after reviewing the stem. This process can be helpful to many successful test takers who might be tempted to make incorrect answer choices fit the stem retrospectively. Note that if you need to add information or change the stem to make an answer choice "fit," it is likely not the correct answer.

Additionally, test takers should realize that sometimes the correct answer to a question is not what they think is the most appropriate answer to a question. Test takers must assume that there is a "best" answer to each question, even though it may not be what they perceive to be the most appropriate answer. Timing oneself with practice questions is good preparation for a successful outcome on a standardized test such as this certification exam. The following section contains examples of challenging questions that may require some extra attention to answer correctly.

Clues to Memorizing Information

When reviewing content before taking an exam, it is helpful to use certain methods of remembering information. For example, remembering the three Ps that indicate the three most common manifestations of diabetes mellitus— polydipsia = extreme thirst, polyuria = frequent urination, and polyphagia = extreme hunger—will assist in answering some questions. The following example illustrates the usefulness of the memorization technique of mnemonics.

EXAMPLE

A 77-year-old woman is taking a medication with strong anticholinergic side effects. She is likely to experience which of the following symptoms?

a. Polyuria and polyphagia

b. Confusion and constipation

c. Hypoglycemia and hypotension

d. Urticaria and difficulty sleeping

Rationale for the correct answer—b: This is pure recall. It needs to be memorized by applying the information to a framework that you can remember. For some students it may be easy to remember the A, B, C, Ds of anticholinergic medications: **a**norexia, **b**lurry vision, **c**onstipation and **c**onfusion, **d**ry mouth, **s**edation and urinary stasis. Sometimes test takers are easily drawn to answers that they are unfamiliar with. In this example, a test taker might choose "c" because it sounds like a reasonable answer and they might simply assume that they had forgotten those side effects. Remember, it is often better to try to think of an answer before reading the answer choices.

Two Different Ideas in One Question

It is important to understand how some answer options contain two phrases or thoughts. These options really are sentences with two distinct points. Usually, the two phrases are connected by *and* or *but*. *Both* of these phrases *must* be true in order for this two-component answer option to be the correct one. One might be tempted to select a longer answer option, such as in the example that follows. However, the length of the answer choice does not indicate that it is the best answer. Be sure to look out for key words in the stem such as *except, always, must, never, avoid, not, more or less likely, best,* and *first*.

EXAMPLE

An older adult experiencing an infection may be *less likely* than a younger person to present with:

a. Fever, leukocytosis

b. Confusion, weakness

c. New onset of incontinence

d. Signs and symptoms of an infection do not change with age

Rationale for the correct answer—a. An older adult would be less likely to experience a fever or an increase in white blood cell count (leukocytosis) than a younger person would. The older adult would be more likely to present with b. Confusion and weakness, or c. New onset of incontinence. The last answer, d., is not true. Older adults often manifest the signs and symptoms of an infection differently than younger people do.

Prioritizing

EXAMPLE

You are receiving reports from the night-shift nurse about the following patients. Which patient demands your immediate attention?

a. An 87-year-old woman with a history of congestive heart failure, now experiencing bilateral pedal edema.

b. A 72-year-old man with a history of hypertension and a morning blood pressure of 130/80.

c. An 81-year-old man with a history of hypertension with new onset of unilateral facial drooping.

d. A 90-year-old woman with pain and stiffness in the distal interphalangeal joints.

Rationale for the correct answer—c: You should recognize that new-onset unilateral facial drooping is a sign of a stroke, and requires immediate intervention. These types of questions can be difficult, because as a nurse each of these patients will need to be assessed during your shift, and it can be hard to select which is the priority patient. In addition, it may be tempting to add or change information. For example, what if the patient with congestive heart failure is now also experiencing shortness of breath? Shouldn't we peek in her room on the way to see our stroke patient? Remember, it is important to stick to the information that is presented when selecting among the answer choices.

CONCLUSIONS

Having reviewed these hints for analyzing questions and being aware of the most common comorbidities that older adults experience, it is recommended that readers review the content and answer the questions following each content area in the following chapters of this review book. Then it is a good idea to visit the ANCC website (http://www.nursecredentialing.org) and take the practice exam. Reviewing content that you have trouble with on the practice test will improve your ability to succeed on the gerontological nurse certification exam.

3

The Aging Population

DEMOGRAPHICS

- The average life span in the United States is close to 79 years of age. Women live an average of 81 years and men an average of 76 years (World Bank Group, 2014).

- There are significant racial disparities in life expectancy. Although White Americans have a life expectancy of 78.8 years, Black Americans live an average of 74.5 years (Arias, 2014).

- Individuals aged 75 years can be expected to live an average of 11 more years, for a total of 86 years (http://www.health.gov/healthypeople).

- Older adults currently represent approximately 13% of the population. By the year 2030, they are expected to represent approximately 21% of the population.

- Older women outnumber older men. Approximately 47% of women 75 and older live alone.

- The increase in the number of older adults in the United States is known as the graying of America.

- The graying of America raises several questions, including:

  - How will a society view a majority comprised of older adults?

  - Will resources be available, such as health care and housing, for older adults to live healthy and happy lives?

- Many older adults may have several chronic medical illnesses that have the potential to

  - Reduce quality of life

  - Increase health care costs

CATEGORIES OF AGING

Some authors have proposed diving older adults into different categories. The rationale behind the categories is to help understand that there is a great diversity in ages included in the term "older adult." Effective nursing care will recognize the unique differences present in each stage of older adulthood and provide a more individualized approach. Indeed, there is as great a difference between a 20-year-old and a 40-year-old as there is between a 65-year-old and an 85-year-old. One proposed subdivision is as follows:

■ Adults aged 65 to 75 are the young-old.

■ Adults aged 75 to 85 are the old-old.

■ Those aged 85 and older are the oldest old.

■ Those who are 100 years and older are centenarians.

■ Persons living to age 110 and older are supercentenarians.

With the life span continuing to increase, will we need more categories in the future?

People who are currently 65 and older have outlived those in previous generations for several reasons.

■ Immunizations became available to prevent diseases such as measles, mumps, rubella, chicken pox, and polio.

■ Annual influenza vaccination greatly decreased morbidity and mortality related to the flu and prevents complications of pneumonia.

■ Pneumonia vaccination is given to most adults, especially high-risk patients—such as those with chronic obstructive pulmonary disease (COPD) or splenectomies—and heart disease patients.

■ Newer diagnostic techniques assisted in the early detection and treatment of disease.

AGEISM AND MYTHS AMONG NURSES AND OTHER HEALTH CARE STAFF

Ageism is defined as a negative attitude or bias toward older adults resulting in the belief that older people cannot or should not participate in societal activities or be given equal opportunities afforded to others. Ageism results in:

■ Lack of medical care of older adults

■ Decreased access to services

■ Potential for poor communication by health care providers

Older adults challenge ageist attitudes by:

■ Participating in organizations that support older adults, such as AARP and local senior citizens organizations
■ Remaining politically active
■ Giving back to their local communities through volunteer activities
■ Continuing to be active participants in the workforce

Within our culture, there are unspoken myths and biases against older adults. Some are based on misinformation, others on antiquated stereotypes. The foundation for ageism lies in these many myths of aging.

Myth #1: Older adults are of little benefit to society.

- The rate of morbidity among older adults is steadily declining.
- Older adults are also mothers, fathers, grandmothers, grandfathers, aunts, uncles, brothers, sisters, friends, and professionals such as teachers, physicians, nurses, and clergy.
- Older adults are of great benefit to those with whom they maintain relationships and in the roles they serve.
- Older adults are one of the nation's greatest and most underutilized resources in that they make up a large volunteer pool that could save state and government funds in unpaid services.

Myth #2: Older adults don't pull their weight in society.

- Older adults who receive Social Security and Medicare have paid into the system from which they are now drawing.
- Although many older adults retire, many others do not. In 2002, 13.2% of older Americans were working or were actively seeking work. A Gallup poll of 986 older adults reported that only 15% of older adults wished to retire, and the vast majority wanted to work as long as possible.
- Ageism in the workplace or sickness and disability may prevent older adults from working, although they may wish to.
- Older adults are raising their grandchildren in record numbers. Nearly 60% of grandparents have provided childcare to their grandchildren in the past or are currently doing so.

Myth #3: Older adults are cranky and disagreeable.

- The continuity theory supports the idea that individuals will move through their later years using personality and coping strategies used previously to maintain stability throughout life. When patients (both young and old) are moved from their homes into institutional settings, it is a healthy coping strategy to attempt to maintain some control over their environment. Older adults may express preferences about when they eat, sleep, and bathe and the foods they prefer. Although some nurses may find these

these choices by creating systems of care that allow flexibility in hospital and nursing home routines.

Myth #4: You can't teach old dogs new tricks.

• Older adults are increasingly returning to school and enhancing their level of education. Many colleges and universities offer older adults the opportunity to attend classes for little or no charge.

• Older adults are never too old to make healthy lifestyle changes in order to improve their overall health and safety.

• Keeping intellectually active is regarded as a hallmark of successful aging.

Myth #5: Older adults are all senile.

• Age-related memory impairments affect a minority of older adults. Estimates of this condition vary considerably, from 7% to 38%.

• The development of dementia is not a normal change of aging, but a pathological disease process evolving from neurological, vascular, infectious, metabolic, or degenerative processes or through trauma. New onset of confusion in older adults can be a sign of infection or an indication of delirium. A rapid onset of cognitive impairment requires diagnostic evaluation.

• Dementia is a chronic loss of cognitive function that is typically gradual in onset and progresses over a long period of time.

• Alzheimer's disease is the most common form of dementia among older adults, making up about half of all dementia diagnoses.

• There are approximately 4.5 million U.S. residents with Alzheimer's disease.

Myth #6: Depression is a normal response to the many losses older adults experience with aging.

• Depression is a treatable medical condition experienced by young and old alike.

• Recent research on depression indicates that there is more to the development of depression than the experience of loss.

• Depression rates are highest among older adults with coexisting medical conditions. Conditions that have a high rate of associated depression include cardiovascular disease, COPD, stroke, and Parkinson's disease. In addition, patients who experience chronic pain as well as older adults living in nursing homes experience higher than average rates of depression.

Myth #7: Older adults are no longer interested in sex.

• Because sexuality is mainly considered a young person's activity—often associated with reproduction—society doesn't usually associate older adults with sex.

• Recent surveys have shown that approximately 30% of older adults had participated in sexual activity within the past month.

• Nurses and other health care providers do a poor job assessing sexual

- Reasons for nurses' lack of attention to the sexuality of older adults include lack of knowledge as well as general inexperience and discomfort.

Myth #8: Most older adults live in nursing homes.

- The majority of older adults live at home and/or alone.
- Less than 5% of people older than 65 years live in a nursing home.

Myth #9: The secret to successful aging is to choose your parents wisely.

- This phrase from the popular work of Rowe and Kahn (1998) on successful aging leads society to believe that little can be done to slow the aging process because it is all set out in an unmodifiable genetic plan dictated by lineage.
- Although genetics are responsible for some parts of the aging process, they become less and less important as older adults age.
- The role of environment and health behaviors significantly replaces the role of genetics in determining the onset of normal and pathological aging.
- Rowe and Kahn (1998) report that approximately one third of physical aging and half of cognitive function is a result of genetic input from parental influences. That leaves two thirds of physical aging and half of cognitive function to be influenced by environmental factors and health behaviors.
- Many older adults, especially centenarians (those who have reached the age of 100), report that the key to successful aging is to enjoy and get satisfaction from life.

Myth #10: When an older adult becomes seriously ill, there is "nothing more that can be done."

- This myth often leads health care professionals to offer less aggressive treatment for disease and to neglect essential components of end-of-life care for older adults.
- While death among older adults may occur after a long life, older adults are not necessarily psychologically prepared for it.
- The end of life is a difficult time for many older adults, but it also presents the opportunity to complete important developmental tasks of aging.
- Nurses can play an important role in helping older adults to complete these developmental tasks, which can make the difference between a good and a bad death.

AGING THEORIES

Several categories of theories have been developed to describe why people age. Biological theories explain that the reason people age and die is because of changes in the human body (e.g., the Hayflick theory). Biological theories include

Biological Theories

Stochastic theories

■ DNA error

■ Accumulation of free radicals

■ Protein cross-linkage

■ Wear and tear

■ Error theory

Nonstochastic theories

■ Gene/biological clock theory

■ Programmed theory

■ Immunity theory

■ Neuroendocrine theory

Generally speaking, stochastic theories point to individual events that happen over the course of a lifetime that accumulate and cause random damage. Nonstochastic theories tend to point to aging as genetically predetermined.

Psychological theories support the idea that an older adult's life ends when he or she has reached all of his or her developmental milestones. Psychological theories of aging include:

■ Maslow's—self-actualization

■ Jung's—self-realization

■ Erikson's—integrity versus despair

Moral/spiritual theories support the idea that once an older individual finds spiritual wholeness, this transcends the need to inhabit a body, and he or she dies. These theories include:

■ Tornstam's theory of gerotranscendence

■ Kohlberg's theory of self-transcendence

Sociological theories explain that when an older adult's usefulness in roles and relationships ends, death occurs.

■ *Disengagement theory* explains that as relationships change or end for older adults, through the process of retirement, disability, or death, a gradual withdrawing of the older adult is evidenced. Less engagement in relationships and social activities is seen, and although new relationships may be formed, these relationships are not as integral to life as previously necessary.

■ *Activity theory* indicates that social activity is an essential component of successful aging. When social activity is halted because of death of loved ones, changes in relationships, or illness and disabilities that affect relationships, aging is accelerated and death becomes nearer.

■ *Continuity theory* proposes that people who age most successfully carry forward the habits, preferences, lifestyles, and relationships from midlife into later life and predicts strategies people will use to progress into old age.

■ *Subculture theory* is the idea that older adults will meaningfully disengage from society in order to create a subculture of people who share common backgrounds and life experiences.

■ *Age stratification theory* suggests that there are social pressures for people to fit into predetermined ideas about how people should act and behave at certain ages.

Family Theory

Family theory provides a framework for understanding human behavior and improving relationships in order to assist individuals, families, communities, and organizations work through major life issues. In older adulthood, major life transitions include:

■ Retirement

■ Relocation

■ Loss of spouse and other family members and friends

■ Financial constraints

Effectively functioning families with good communication are critical to helping older adults make transitions smoothly and decreasing the risk of depression and other negative effects of stress. Poorly functioning family processes leave older adults at risk for ineffective coping. These families may benefit from family therapy as well as individual therapy. Key family theories include those of Freud and Bowen.

Motivational Theory

Motivational theory is generally associated with workplace employment and the desire to develop more effective employees.

■ Herzberg's hygienic needs theory focuses on the need to avoid discomfort and achieve personal fulfillment through maintaining good relationships, work conditions, salary, status, security, and a satisfying personal life. People will be more motivated to do a good job if their comfort needs are met.

■ McGregor's X–Y theory focuses on whether people are lazy or ambitious.

■ Adams's equity theory focuses on patterns of fairness.

■ McClelland's motivational theory centers on motivational power.

In relation to older adults, motivational theory can be more specifically applied to changes in behaviors needed to improve health, for example:

■ Smoking cessation

■ Alcohol withdrawal and abstention

■ Nutritional changes

■ Weight loss

■ Exercise

■ Sleep hygiene

Motivational theories support the idea that it is critical to determine one's motivational factor in order to change behavior. Thus, the determination of a critical end result and continuous feedback toward that result are important factors in changing health behaviors among older adults. Researchers in motivational theory have identified the following potential motivators.

■ Desire to avoid a negative result of one's behavior

■ Achievement of a goal

■ Recognition of activity

■ The rewards of health behavior itself

■ Responsibility

■ Advancement or progress

■ Personal growth

Health-promotion activities may be centered on these potential motivators to enhance compliance and success.

COMMUNICATION WITH OLDER ADULTS

Communication with older adult clients is often complicated by many factors. Some factors that may result in a nursing diagnosis of impaired communication include:

■ Different languages

■ Hard of hearing

■ Dysphagia

■ Dementia

In working with older adults, effective communication is essential and is the responsibility of the health care provider. Outcomes of successful

■ The client being able to communicate effectively with health care providers

■ The client utilizing alternative communication methods to convey his or her meaning

■ The client being able to correctly understand messages conveyed by health care providers

Interventions used to aid in effective communication include:

■ Assessing the client's receptive abilities—can the older adult understand what you are communicating?

■ Assessing the client's expressive abilities—can the older adult communicate his or her needs and desires?

■ Identifying the client's sensory impairments that affect his or her communication, such as

  • Hearing impairments

  • Aphasias

  • Visual impairments

■ Facing the client directly and speaking slowly, clearly, and concisely

■ Demonstrating the skill or activity that you would like to communicate to the older adult

■ Using interpreter services as necessary

■ Using paper, pencil, or computer communication when necessary

■ Validating the client's understanding of messages by asking him or her to repeat what was said

■ Being alert for nonverbal signs of behavior, especially in cognitively impaired older adults

■ Providing the older adult with yes/no choices

■ Providing easy instructions in short, simple sentences

■ Using physical cues and gesturing

■ Limiting choices to reduce confusion

The Alzheimer's Association (2014) recommends a number of assessment questions and communication tips, which are displayed in Table 3.1. Assessment of specific receptive and expressive abilities is needed in order to understand the patient's communication difficulties and facilitate communication.

TEACHING–LEARNING THEORIES AND PRINCIPLES

Teaching refers to transference of knowledge, and learning results from an educational experience aimed at improving knowledge and skills or changing

TABLE 3.1   Tools to Assess Language Deficits and Facilitate Communication

ASSESS RECEPTIVE ABILITIES	HOW TO FACILITATE COMMUNICATION
Can the patient understand a yes/no choice?	Ask simple, direct questions that require only a *yes* or *no* response.
Can the patient read simple instructions?	Provide instructions in a place that is easily visible to the patient.
Can the patient understand simple verbal instructions?	Use short, simple sentences. Use one-step instructions to enhance the individual's ability to process—for example, it's time to wash [smile; pause]; I will help you [pause and proceed]. Avoid slang, idioms, and nuances.
Can the patient understand instructions given with physical cues?	Use gestures. Model the desired behavior (e.g., eating). Be sensitive to the fact that, although the person may not understand words, he or she often can read your body language, sincerity, and mood.
Can the patient make a choice when presented with two objects or options?	Limit choices; too many options will cause confusion and frustration.

ASSESS EXPRESSIVE ABILITIES	HOW TO FACILITATE COMMUNICATION
Does the patient have difficulty finding the correct word?	If you are sure of the word the person is trying to say, repeat it. If you are not sure, then don't guess, because that will increase the person's confusion and frustration.
Does the patient have difficulty creating sentences or a logical flow of ideas?	Listen for meaningful words and ideas. Try to identify the key thoughts and ideas. Do not dismiss a person as "totally confused."
Does the patient curse, use offensive or aggressive language, or exhibit aggressive or combative behaviors?	Don't reprimand. Respond to the emotion, not the words. Validate feelings. Assess for unmet needs, including those related to misperceptions, hunger, thirst, toileting needs, pain, and so on.
Does the patient avoid verbalization altogether or mutter meaninglessly in various tones?	Read nonverbal communication. Anticipate needs.

GENERAL COMMUNICATION TIPS

- ▨ If the patient's primary language is not English, determine whether he or she can communicate more effectively in another language; ask the family; and use an interpreter if necessary.
- ▨ Identify hearing and vision impairments; ask about prior use of assistive devices (hearing aids and glasses) and assure use of these devices in the hospital.
- ▨ Reduce environmental distractions that compete for attention when conversing with the patient.

(continued)

TABLE 3.1 Tools to Assess Language Deficits and Facilitate Communication (*continued*)

■ Approach the patient from the front, make eye contact, address the person by name, and speak in a calm voice.

■ Talk first; pause; touch second, reducing the person's sense of threat.

■ Avoid verbal testing or questioning beyond the person's capacity.

■ Avoid using the in-room intercom, which may confuse and frighten the patient.

■ Do not argue or insist that the patient accept your reality.

■ Be aware of memory impairments in addition to communication difficulties. For example, if a patient's short-term memory is less than a few minutes, it is dangerous to leave the patient alone even if he or she seems to understand the direction, "wait here." Likewise, it is unwise to expect the patient to use a call light to get help. For patients with very impaired short-term memory, each encounter with a staff member may be perceived as the first encounter, even if the staff member just left the room and returned a few minutes later.

Adapted from the Alzheimer's Association (2014).

feedback of good behaviors implemented as a result of the teaching–learning process. Negative behaviors associated with the process are ignored. Practicing the right behavior repeatedly is critical.

Cognitive teaching–learning theories focus on an active learning approach aimed at developing human insight. Goal setting and attainment are the underlying principles of this teaching–learning process.

Constructivist theories surround an engaging process that combines both behaviorist and cognitive strategies to promote effective teaching and learning. The foundation for learning is built on students' past experiences.

■ Although many myths of aging lead health care providers to avoid teaching in this population, older adults are capable of gaining new knowledge and changing behaviors even at very advanced ages.

■ Older adults have many heterogeneous educational experiences and learning styles that require individualization of teaching strategies.

■ Identifying an older adult's learning style and individualizing one's teaching methods accordingly are important for successful teaching and learning to take place.

■ Health literacy is defined as the degree to which an individual has the capacity to obtain, process, and understand basic health information and services necessary to make appropriate health care decisions.

■ Low health literacy occurs frequently in older adults, who also tend to be those most in need of health services. Health literacy requires that older adults not only be able to read information—and to understand what they are reading—hear instructions, calculate medications, and communicate questions.

■ Low health literacy often impacts the ability of older adults to fully understand medication instructions and health interventions.

■ Low health literacy disrupts a client's ability to effectively prepare for diagnostic tests, make follow-up appointments, and maintain health.

■ Health literacy is a significant factor in noncompliance with health care treatments and medications.

■ Clear communication has the capacity to assist those with low health literacy to maintain health.

GERONTOLOGICAL NURSING TODAY

With the increased population of older adults, there is a great need to increase the number of competent geriatric-educated nurses. Although nursing was the first profession to develop standards of gerontological care and provide a certification mechanism to ensure competence, gerontological nursing has been slow to gain recognition as a nursing specialty. Although an increase in the number of nursing programs offer courses in geriatric nursing or integrate best geriatric nursing practices throughout programs, geriatric nursing is still not a popular specialty area among nursing students.

Some of the terms associated with nursing and the elderly are used interchangeably.

■ *Geriatric nursing* refers to the nursing care of older people with health problems or those requiring tertiary care.

■ *Gerontological nursing* includes health promotion, education, and disease prevention (primary and secondary care).

■ *Gerontic nursing*, although not a commonly known term, encompasses both of these aspects of nursing care of older adults.

The American Nurses Association first recognized geriatric nursing as a specialty in 1966. Standards to guide the practice of gerontological nursing were first published by the American Nurses Association in 1976 and later revised in 1987, 1995, and 2010. Several organizations specialize in geriatric nursing.

■ The National Gerontological Nursing Organization was developed in 1984 to support the growth of knowledge related to gerontological nursing science.

■ The Gerontological Society of America, the American Society of Aging, and the American Geriatrics Society are multidisciplinary organizations that support aging knowledge and research.

REFERENCES

Alzheimer's Association. (2014). *Tips for better communication*. Retrieved from https://www.alz.org/national/documents/brochure_communication.pdf

Arias, E. (2014). United States life tables, 2009. *National vital statistics reports* (vol. 62

Hartford Institute for Geriatric Nursing. (2012). *Try this: Best practices in nursing care to older adults*. New York, NY: Author. Retrieved from http://www.hartfordign.org

National Association of Child Care Resources and Referral Associates. (2008). Grandparents: A critical childcare safety net. Retrieved from http://www.naccrra.org/sites/default/files/default_site_pages/2011/2008_grandparents_report-finalrept_0.pdf

Rowe, J., & Kahn, S. (1996). Successful aging. *Gerontologist. 37 (4)* 433–440.

World Bank Group (2014). *Life expectancy world populations*. Retrieved from http://www.naccrra.org/sites/default/files/default_site_pages/2011/2008_grandparents_report-finalrept_0.pdf

4

Assessment

HISTORY AND PHYSICAL EXAM CONSIDERATIONS

Health History

The health assessment always begins by taking a health history. This usually is the first meeting between the older adult and the nurse, and it marks the beginning of the therapeutic relationship. A sufficient amount of time should be set aside for taking the health history so a complete and accurate history may be obtained. Older adults may have difficulty extracting dates and details about a health history that extends over many decades, and which may include numerous health care encounters. There are many other barriers to getting a detailed and complete healthy history from older adults, including:

- Age (older adults have a longer story to tell)
- Reliance on memory for complicated details, including lab changes and medications
- Tendency to underreport, especially when rushed
- Communication difficulties (nurses should check to see whether dentures and hearing aids, if needed, are in place and functioning prior to the patient interview)

It is important to allow patients time to reflect on their health history and support them with questions that will aid in remembering details about former medical and surgical events. Older adults may choose to withhold certain medical information from the interviewer because:

- The information may be too upsetting or difficult to discuss.
- The client may fear the consequences of his or her health problems. Memories of painful tests or the fear of a stressful diagnosis may cause the older adult to minimize symptoms.

- The client may fear being a burden on the health care provider or on his or her children and thus hide or minimize symptoms of disease.
- The older adult may consider important and treatable indicators of disease to be normal and expected changes of aging.

A health history includes:

- Past medical history
- Past surgical history
- Cultural background
- Sources of social support
- Sources of financial support
- Occupation/retirement status
- Education
- Living arrangements
- Health-promotion behaviors
  - Smoking
  - Alcohol use
  - Sleep patterns
  - Diet (use 24-hour recall)
  - Exercise
  - Use of herbal supplements
  - Stress management
- Medications (including herbals and over-the-counter medications)
- Presence of common problems of aging
  - Dementia
  - Depression
  - Musculoskeletal disorders (osteoarthritis)
  - Sensory changes
  - Urinary function
  - Health literacy

Conduct a thorough review of systems.

- Cardiovascular system
- Respiratory system
- Peripheral vascular system

■ Integumentary system

■ Gastrointestinal system

■ Genitourinary system

■ Musculoskeletal system (ambulation)

■ Neurologic system (including senses)

Assess function and cognition as precipitating symptoms of illness in older adults.

■ A sudden decline in functional status or a change in ability to independently complete activities of daily living (bathing, dressing, toileting, eating, transferring, and ambulating) often signals the onset of physiological disease among older adults. The Katz Index (Katz, Dow, Cash, & Grotz, 1970) is a highly regarded functional assessment tool used widely in many health care settings to assess function among older adults.

■ Acute change in cognitive status, known as delirium, may be the first presenting sign of illness among older adults. This is true for both cognitively intact and cognitively impaired older adults. Because altered cognitive status is one of the more commonly occurring symptoms of disease among older adults, cognitive assessment using a valid and reliable instrument, such as the Mini-Cog, is appropriate (see Figure 4.1).

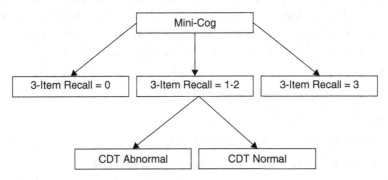

FIGURE 4.1   The Mini-Cog and Mini-Cog scoring algorithm.

Administration of the Mini-Cog is as follows.

1. Instruct the patient to listen carefully and remember three unrelated words and then to repeat the words.

2. Instruct the patient to draw the face of a clock, either on a blank sheet of paper or on a sheet with the clock circle already drawn on the page. After the patient puts the numbers on the clock face, ask him or her to draw the hands of the clock to read a specific time (clock-draw test [CDT]).

3. Ask the patient to repeat the three previously stated words.

   Scoring

1. Give 1 point for each recalled word after the CDT distractor.
2. Patients recalling none of the three words are classified as demented (score = 0).
3. Patients recalling all three words are classified as nondemented (score = 3).
4. Patients with intermediate word recall of one or two words are classified based on the CDT (abnormal = demented; normal = nondemented).
5. The CDT is normal if all numbers are present in the correct sequence and position, and the hands readably display the requested time.

Source: From Borson, Scanlan, Brush, Vitallano, and Dokmak (2000). Copyright John Wiley & Sons Limited. Reproduced with permission.

Physical Assessment

Following the health history and a complete review of systems, a head-to-toe physical examination should be conducted. This is how objective data are obtained to form diagnoses. Evaluate the patient's vital signs.

■ Temperature—response to infection among older adults varies greatly; some older adults respond to infections with elevated temperatures, whereas others with aggressive infections may show no febrile response. The fever response may be blunted among older adults because of:
  • Diminished production and reduced response of pyrogens
  • Lower baseline temperature
  • Impaired immunity
  • Impaired ability to regulate heat and cold
  • Delayed onset of fever when infection is present
■ Pulse between 60 and 100 beats per minute—note irregular rhythms and follow up with electrocardiogram testing, if necessary
■ Respiration (12–18 breaths per minute)
■ Measurements of height, weight, and body mass index (BMI) are essential to developing a baseline for further comparison of nutritional and hydration levels and bone loss. BMIs of less than 25 are considered ideal. BMI parameters are:
  • Below 18.5 = underweight
  • Between 18.5 and 24.9 = normal
  • 25 to 29.9 = overweight
  • 30 and above = obese

■ Blood pressure should be evaluated in the sitting, immediate standing, and 1-minute standing positions, especially if the older adult is taking antihypertensive medications. Decreases in blood pressure of over 20 mmHg indicate orthostatic hypertension and require further evaluation. Blood pressure readings should follow the Eighth Report of the Joint National Committee on Prevention, Detection, Evaluation, and Treatment of High Blood Pressure (JNC-VIII) blood pressure guidelines (see Table 4.1). It is helpful to remember the following basic strategies for hypertension management.

• Assess and manage blood pressure before it gets too high

• In people older than age 50, systolic blood pressure is important and should be managed effectively

• Two or more antihypertensive medications are often necessary to maintain control

• Continued evaluation is often necessary, so maintenance of the therapeutic nurse–client relationship is essential

• The most recent treatment goals for people 60 years of age and older are to maintain a systolic blood pressure of less than 150 and a diastolic blood pressure of less than 90. This represents a relaxation of the previous JNC-VII management goals.

TABLE 4.1   JNC-VIII Blood Pressure Guidelines

BLOOD PRESSURE CLASSIFICATION	SYSTOLIC BLOOD PRESSURE (mmHG)		DIASTOLIC BLOOD PRESSURE (mmHG)
Normal	< 120	and	< 80
Prehypertensive	120–139	or	80–89
Stage I hypertension	140–159	or	90–99
Stage II hypertension	> 160	or	> 100

From U.S. Department of Health and Human Services, National Institutes of Health, National Heart, Lung, and Blood Institute, National High Blood Pressure Education Program (2014).

In addition to vital signs, the head-to-toe physical assessment includes an evaluation of the following systems.

■ Skin

• Hemangiomas

• Liver spots

• Harmless senile lentigines

• Inflamed skin tags (skin projections)

• Keratoses, precancerous, and cancerous lesions

- Herpes zoster
- Decubitus ulcers
- Dryness
- Unexplained bruises or cuts

■ Hair growth and nails
  - Uniformity
  - Diminished hair growth
  - Fungal infections of the nails

■ Head and neck
  - Lesions or trauma
  - Evaluate the sclera for whiteness
  - Note the arcus senilis (grayish arc surrounding the cornea and caused by lipid deposits on the cornea, not necessarily associated with high blood cholesterol)
  - Visual acuity
  - Central vision (ability to see fine details, read, recognize faces)
  - Evaluate for signs and symptoms that may indicate cataracts and macular degeneration (the leading cause of vision loss among older adults) and refer to an ophthalmologist for follow-up of abnormal findings
  - Identify the tympanic membrane and light reflex in the ear
  - Palpate nose for tenderness and signs and symptoms of infection
  - Evaluate mouth and teeth for deviations from normal and referrals made to a dentist for further management of mouth and tooth disorders
  - Palpate thyroid gland for enlargement and nodules

■ Heart and lungs
  - Evaluate the carotid arteries and jugular veins in the neck—they should be symmetrical, nonbounding, nondistended, and absent of bruits and adventitious sounds
  - Inspect and auscultate the heart beginning at the apex. The first two heart sounds should be auscultated, and any adventitious sounds, murmurs, rhythms, and pulsations should be noted
  - Murmurs (defective heart values) may be innocent (no associated signs/symptoms) or may be associated with
    - Shortness of breath (SOB)
    - Enlarged neck veins
    - Dyspnea, perspiration on minimal exertion

■ Inspect lungs and palpate for tactile fremitus and equal expansion

■ Percuss lung fields for areas of hyperresonance or dullness

■ Assess peripheral pules, warmth and color in extremities

■ Musculoskeletal system

- Assess ambulation

- Assess joint range of motion, tenderness, crepitus

- Begin at temporomandibular joint and proceed inferiorally to the ankles and feet

- Evaluate each joint, bone, and muscle group for abnormalities, tenderness, bilateral equalness, strength, and range of motion

■ Abdomen

- Check for abnormal scars, pulsations, or distention

- Auscultate bowel sounds in all four quadrants

■ Genitourinary

- Older women should continue to see a gynecologist for evaluation of breast and gynecological disorders common with aging

- Older men should undergo an annual examination for prostate enlargement or malignancies

■ Laboratory tests

- Proper use of laboratory tests in evaluating older adults requires both knowledge of the normal ranges for age and the nurses' awareness of clients' health and medication history

- Laboratory tests commonly used in assessing older adults are provided in Table 4.2

TABLE 4.2   Common Laboratory Tests Used to Assess Older Adults

---

Cholesterol: Total cholesterol (TC), high-density lipoprotein (HDL), and low-density lipoprotein (LDL)

Normal Ranges

TC < 200 mg/dL
HDL > 45 mg/dL = lower risk of cardiovascular disease (CVD)
LDL < 100 mg/dL = goal
Tests the amount of circulating cholesterol levels. Good indicator for risk of CVD, as well as to manage medications to prevent hyperlipidemia. There can be some variability in goal ranges

Complete blood count (CBC), hemoglobin (Hg), hematocrit (Hct), and white blood cells (WBCs)

Normal Ranges

Men
Hg: 13–18 g/dL
Hct: 45%–52%

Women
Hg: 12–16 g/dL
Hct: 37%–48%
WBCs: 4,300–10,800 cells/mm^3

(continued)

TABLE 4.2   Common Laboratory Tests Used to Assess Older Adults (*continued*)

Tests for red blood cell (Hg, Hct, erythrocyte sedimentation rate) function and WBC function (leukocytes) to determine the ability of red blood cells to carry oxygen and WBC's role in infection. These reference ranges may tend to be lower in older adults. Hg may be as low as 9 in women and 10 in men, and Hct may be as low as 35% in women and 38% in men. These results can also be chronically elevated for patients with chronic obstructive pulmonary disease or other chronic impairments in pulmonary function.

Drug assays (e.g., digoxin, dilantin, phenytoin, theophylline, lithium)
See individual tests for reference ranges
A collection of tests used to measure the level of certain medications in the body; helpful in management of medication dosing

Glucose and hemoglobin A1C (HgA1C)
Normal Ranges
Glucose (fasting) < 100
HgA1C < 7%
Used to evaluate blood sugar levels and effectiveness of glucose-management medications on glucose function among older adults; HgA1C recommendations may be relaxed to < 8% for frail older adults

Iron (Fe)
Normal Range
Serum iron 35–165 mcg/L
Plays a role in Hg and red blood cell function. Low iron is diagnostic for iron-deficiency anemia

International normalized ratio (INR)
Normal Range
0.9–1.1
Normal INR range for patients on anticoagulant therapy 2–3.5
Tests body's clotting ability. Often used to evaluate response to warfarin therapy

Kidney function tests (BUN) and creatinine (CR)
Normal Ranges
BUN 10–20 mg/dL
Men
Serum CR: 0.6–1.2 mg/dL
Women
Serum CR: 0.5–1.1 mg/dL
Commonly used to evaluate kidney function among older adults

Liver function tests
See individual tests for reference ranges
Used to evaluate normal and pathological liver functioning

Thyroid function tests (T3, T4, TSH)
Normal Ranges
T3: 75–220 ng/dL
T4: 4.5–11.2 mcg/dL
TSH: 0.4–4.2 uU/mL
Because thyroid problems are prevalent among older adults, these tests are frequently used to determine thyroid function

Vitamin assays
See individual tests for reference ranges
Tests for function of vitamins in the body, such as vitamin D. Vitamins play an essential role in all bodily system functions

NORMAL AGING CHANGES

Normal changes of aging are sometimes considered to be inevitable and irreversible. However, a great deal of variability in the age-related changes occur among older adults. Individual aging is influenced by many factors that are both preventable and reversible. It is of critical importance for nurses to understand the normal physiological changes associated with aging. Nurses will be capable of differentiating these changes from abnormal or pathological organ system changes. These changes are discussed, as well as necessary nursing interventions.

Cardiovascular System

■ The heart becomes larger and occupies more space in the chest

■ Cardiac output declines

■ More adventitious S4 heart sounds are evident

■ Premature contractions and arrhythmias may occur

■ Wounds heal more slowly due to diminished blood flow

■ Decreases in cardiac function can impact the distribution, breakdown, and excretion of drugs

■ Older adults often experience a low diastolic blood pressure

■ Older adults often experience an increased pulse pressure

■ Although changes may be normal, they may also indicate cardiomyopathy, which warrants further cardiovascular assessment

■ Provide patient teaching regarding the role of exercise to ultimately reduce strain on the heart and blood pressure

■ Heart murmurs (S4) may require further tests to determine their effect

■ Fatigue, SOB and dyspnea on exertion, dizziness, chest pain, headache, sudden weight gain, and changes in cognitive function or cognition require full assessment

■ Low diastolic pressure (in addition to high diastolic pressure) is a risk factor for cerebrovascular accidents or strokes

Peripheral Vascular System

■ Increase in the peripheral vascular resistance (blood has a hard time returning to the heart and lungs)

■ Valves in the veins do not function efficiently and form (nonpathological) edema

■ Monitor older adults' cholesterol levels with lowering agents to prevent atherosclerosis and arteriosclerosis

■ Inform patients that exercise can lower cholesterol levels

■ Discuss the right medication, exercise program, and diet for the patient as a means to slow the progression of cardiac changes

Respiratory System

■ Vital respiratory capacity decreases

■ Lungs lose elasticity

■ Loss of water and calcium in bones causes the thoracic cage to stiffen

■ Amount of cilia lining system decreases

■ Cough reflex decreases

■ Auscultating sounds is difficult as lung sounds may be diminished, so ausculation must be done on all lung fields in a quiet environment

■ Implement interventions for older adults at risk for choking; patients with ill-fitting dentures as well as those who have previously had a stroke are at increased risk

■ Encourage regular exercise

Integumentary System

■ Skin becomes thinner and more fragile

■ Skin is dry and loses elasticity (wrinkles)

■ Sweat gland production lessens, which leads to less perspiration

■ Subcutaneous fat and muscular layers diminish, which results in less padding and bruising more easily

■ Dryness is common

■ There is an increased risk of skin tears

■ Fingernails and toenails may become thicker and more brittle

■ Hair may become gray, fine, and thin

■ Facial hair may develop on women

■ Body hair decreases on men and women

■ Promote the use of sun block, and tell patients to avoid overexposure to sun

■ Older adults should avoid the use of soaps that dry the skin and use lotion after bathing

■ Older adults with limitations in mobility should protect high-risk areas, such as elbows and heels, with padding

■ Refer diabetic patients to podiatrists for routine foot care

Gastrointestinal System

■ Decreased peristalsis of esophagus makes food more difficult to swallow; tooth loss is not considered a normal change of aging

■ Decreased gut motility, gastric acid production, and absorption of nutrients

Urinary System

■ Kidneys experience a loss of nephrons and glomeruli

■ Bladder tone and volume capacity decrease

■ Incontinence is not a normal aging change but often occurs in response to normal changes. These normal changes can include a decrease in bladder capacity and a decrease in muscle tone. Types of urinary incontinence include:

  • Stress

  • Urge

  • Overflow

  • Transient

■ Risk factors for incontinence include:

  • Immobility

  • Impaired cognition

  • Medication

  • Constipation

  • Diabetes

  • Stroke

Assess for urinary incontinence complications such as:

■ Falls

■ Skin irritation

■ Social isolation

■ Depression

Implement voiding schedules when necessary.

Sexual/Reproductive System

■ There is an overall decrease in testosterone in men, and decreases in estrogen and progesterone in women

■ Conduct sexual assessments

■ Help older adults feel comfortable when discussing sexuality

■ Women
  - Follicular depletion occurs in the ovaries
  - Natural breast tissue is replaced by fatty tissue
  - Labia shrink
  - Vaginal lubrications decrease
  - Shortening and narrowing of the vagina occurs
  - Strength of orgasmic contraction diminishes
  - Orgasmic phase is decreased
  - Artificial vaginal lubricants may help to compensate for normal aging changes

■ Men
  - Increased time may be needed for erections and ejaculation
  - Inform men to increase the time between erections
  - Discuss availability of oral erectile agents

Sensory System

■ Vision
  - Visual acuity declines
  - Ability of pupil to constrict in response to stimuli decreases
  - Peripheral vision declines
  - Presbyopia is common, resulting from a loss of elasticity in the lens of the eye and leading to a decrease in the ability of the lens to refocus on near objects and light
  - Lens of the eye becomes yellow, altering the perception of certain colors
  - Arcus senilis (ring around the cornea) may appear; this has no impact on vision
  - Make sure older adults have a baseline eye assessment early in older adulthood and follow-up eye exams yearly

■ Hearing
  - Amount of hard cerumen increases
  - Presbycusis is common, resulting from a gradual loss of high-frequency sensory neurons that conduct hearing

■ Taste and smell
  - Obtain a thorough history of taste and smell sensations
  - Conduct a physical examination of the nose and mouth
  - Obtain a thorough diet history
  - Implement diet interventions to avoid overcompensation for changes in taste with sweet and salty foods

Neurologic System

■ Mild memory loss is common, but cognitive impairment is not a normal change of aging

■ Help older adults maintain an active body and mind

■ Encourage older adults to participate in activities that stimulate the mind, such as doing crossword puzzles, playing Scrabble, and reading

Immune System

■ The immune system is slower to respond to infection

■ White blood cell (WBC) response may be blunted or absent

■ Autoimmune disorders become more common

REFERENCES

Borson, S., Scanlan, J., Brush, M., Vitallano, P., & Dokmak, A. (2000). The Mini-Cog: A cognitive "vital signs" measure for dementia screening in multi-lingual elderly. *International Journal of Geriatric Psychiatry*, *15*(11), 1021–1027.

Katz, S., Dow, T. D., Cash, H. R., & Grotz, R. C. (1970). Progress in the development of the index of ADL. *The Gerontologist*, *10*(1), 20–30.

U.S. Department of Health and Human Services, National Institutes of Health, National Heart, Lung, and Blood Institute National High Blood Pressure Education Program. (2014). Bethesda, MD: Author.

5

Health Promotion

Pathological changes of aging may result from poor health practices acquired early in life that continue into older adulthood. The Centers for Disease Control (2013) report that between 2007 and 2009 the most common causes of death in the United States were heart disease, cancer, and lower respiratory disease. This disease burden is exacerbated by lifestyle choices that include tobacco use, poor diet, lack of physical activity, alcohol consumption, and microbial agents. Research has demonstrated that older adults benefit from health-promotion activities, even in their later years. In fact, health promotion is as important in older adulthood as it is in childhood. It is never too late to improve nutrition, start exercising, get a better night's sleep, and improve overall health and safety.

LEVELS OF PREVENTION

Primary Prevention

Primary prevention involves *measures to prevent an illness or disease from occurring* and includes:

- Smoking cessation
- Limiting alcohol consumption
- Improving nutrition
- Exercise
- Ensuring adequate sleep
- Promoting safe lifestyles
- Updating immunizations

Secondary Prevention (Screening)

Secondary prevention refers to *methods and procedures to detect the presence of disease* in the early stages so that effective treatment and cure are more likely. Routine mammograms, hypertension screening, and prostate-specific antigen blood tests are a few examples of this type of screening.

Strategies for detecting disease at an early stage involve annual physical examinations; laboratory blood tests for tumor markers, cholesterol, and other highly treatable illnesses; and diagnostic imaging for the presence of internal disease. Secondary disease-specific early detection guidelines are listed in Table 5.1.

Tertiary Prevention (Disease Management)

Tertiary prevention is needed after the disease or condition has been diagnosed and treated in *an attempt to return the client to an optimum level of health and wellness despite the disease or condition.* Physical and occupational therapy and speech pathology services following a cerebrovascular accident are typical examples of tertiary prevention strategies.

BARRIERS TO HEALTH PROMOTION AMONG OLDER ADULTS

- Misconceptions about the benefits of health promotion for older adults
- Separating the normal changes of aging from pathological illness
- Motivation to change (see motivational theories in Chapter 3)
- Lack of reimbursement for health-promotion behavior

Alcohol Use

Alcohol dependence and alcoholism has the potential for negative consequences among older adults, including negative effects on:

- Motor function
- Cognition
- Health
- Quality of life

Alcohol use can be difficult to assess among older adults.

- Symptoms of alcohol use among older adults include alteration in mental status and function, which may mimic the symptoms of delirium, dementia, or depression.
- Older adults are usually no longer in the workforce, where the daily performance failures that are common with alcohol abuse are often detected.

TABLE 5.1 **Secondary Prevention Strategies for Older Adults**

INTERVENTION CONSIDERED AND RECOMMENDED FOR THE PERIODIC HEALTH EXAMINATION	LEADING CAUSE OF DEATH
	Heart diseases
	Malignant neoplasm (lung, colorectal, breast)
	Cerebrovascular diseases
	Chronic obstructive pulmonary diseases
	Pneumonia and influenza

Interventions for the General Population

<u>Screening</u>	<u>Injury prevention</u>
Blood pressure	Lap and shoulder belts
Height and weight	Motorcycle and bicycle helmets[d]
Fecal occult blood test[a] and/or sigmoidoscopy	Fall prevention[d]
Mammogram and clinical breast exam[b] (women < 69 years)	Safe storage or removal of firearms[d]
	Smoke detectors[d]
Pap test (women)	Set hot water heater to 130°F or below[d]
Vision screening	CPR training for household members
Assess for hearing impairment	
Assess for problem drinking	
	<u>Dental health</u>
	Regular visits to dental care provider[d]
	Floss, brush with fluoride toothpaste daily[d]
<u>Counseling</u>	<u>Sexual behavior</u>
Substance use	STD prevention: avoid high-risk sexual behavior[d]; use condoms
Tobacco cessation	
Avoid alcohol/drug use while driving, swimming, boating, etc.[d]	
<u>Diet and exercise</u>	<u>Immunizations</u>
Limit fat and cholesterol; maintain caloric balance; emphasize grains, fruits, vegetables	Pneumococcal vaccine
	Influenza
	Tetanus–diphtheria (Td) boosters
Adequate calcium intake (women)	<u>Chemoprophylaxis</u>
Regular physical activity[d]	Discuss hormone prophylaxis, for menopausal women

Interventions for High-Risk Populations

Institutionalized persons	
Chronic medical conditions: TB contacts; low income; immigrants; alcoholics	PPD: hepatitis A vaccine; amantadine/rimantadine
Persons 75 years or older or persons 70 years and older with risk factors for falls	PPD
	Fall prevention intervention
Cardiovascular disease risk factors	Consider cholesterol screening
Family history of skin cancer; nevi; fair skin, eyes, or hair	Avoid excess and midday sun, use protective clothing[d]
Native Americans/Alaska Natives	PPD: hepatitis A vaccine Hepatitis A
Travelers to developing countries	vaccine; hepatitis B vaccine
Blood-product recipients	HIV screen; hepatitis B vaccine
High-risk sexual behavior	Hepatitis A vaccine; HIV screen; hepatitis B vaccine; RPR/VDRL

(continued)

TABLE 5.1 Secondary Prevention Strategies for Older Adults (*continued*)

INTERVENTION CONSIDERED AND RECOMMENDED FOR THE PERIODIC HEALTH EXAMINATION	LEADING CAUSE OF DEATH
Injection or street drug use	PPD; hepatitis A vaccine; HIV screen; hepatitis B vaccine; RPR/VDRL; advice to reduce infection risk
Health care/lab workers	PPD; hepatitis A vaccine amantadine/ rimantadine; hepatitis B vaccine
Persons susceptible to varicella	Varicella vaccine

Notes: [a] annually; [b] mammogram every 1 to 2 years, mammogram every 1 to 2 years with annual clinical breast exams; [c] all women who have been sexually active and who have a cervix: at least every three years. Consider discontinuation of testing after age 65 if previous regular screening yielded consistently normal results; [d] the ability of clinician counseling to influence this behavior is unproven.

Adapted from the Agency for Healthcare Research and Quality (2014).

Alcoholism is a greater problem for older adults because older adults are not able to physiologically detoxify and excrete alcohol as effectively as younger people. Assessment of alcohol use may be most effectively accomplished using an instrument such as the CAGE questionnaire.

▦ Have you ever tried to **c**ut down on your drinking?

▦ Do you become **a**nnoyed when others ask you about drinking?

▦ Do you ever feel **g**uilty about your drinking?

▦ Do you ever use alcohol in the morning as an **e**ye-opener?

Older adults with alcohol problems who receive treatment can achieve positive health outcomes. In fact, when older adults receive effective treatment for their alcoholism, their prognosis is much better than it is for their younger counterparts. When alcohol abuse is suspected among older adults, it is necessary to refer them immediately to an appropriate program for effective treatment—such as Alcoholics Anonymous or an in- or outpatient detoxification and treatment program. Special treatment considerations should be applied to older adults during acute alcohol withdrawal related to normal and pathological aging changes.

Smoking

Cigarette smoking has multiple harmful effects on older adults, including, but not limited to, cardiovascular and respiratory disease and cancer. The current cohorts of older adults are among the first people who have potentially smoked throughout their entire adult lives. It is possible for older adults to experience the benefits of smoking cessation even in old age. It is important to note that older adults may be more motivated to quit smoking than their younger counterparts because they are likely to experience some of the damage that smoking has caused. Smoking cessation interventions include:

■ Behavioral management classes

■ Support groups

■ Nicotine replacement therapies

■ Antidepression medications (e.g., Wellbutrin)

Nutrition and Hydration

As in younger adults, the diets of older Americans are often suboptimal. The many risk factors for improper nutrition among older adults include the following.

■ Normal changes of aging place older adults at a higher risk for nutritional deficiencies

■ Pathological diseases

■ Decreases in smell, vision, and taste and the high frequency of dental problems

■ Lifelong eating habits, such as a diet high in fat and cholesterol

■ Diminishing senses of taste and smell result in a diminished desire to eat, leading to malnutrition

■ Limited income

■ Lack of transportation to purchase food

■ Social isolation

Failure to thrive (FTT) is a syndrome used to describe clients who experience malnutrition in the absence of an explanatory medical diagnosis. FTT is often found with:

■ Dehydration

■ Impaired cognition

■ Dementia

■ Impaired ambulation

■ Difficulty with at least two activities of daily living

■ Neglect

Nutritional assessment might include:

■ 24-hour recall

■ Nutritional assessment forms (Figure 5.1)

Interventions to promote nutrition include:

■ Patient teaching and reinforcements regarding good nutrition (see Chapter 3 for a discussion of the theories and principles of teaching and learning)

HEALTH PROMOTION

Exercise

The role of regular exercise in promoting health and preventing disease cannot be sufficiently emphasized. Regular exercise results in:

■ Reduced constipation
■ Improved sleep
■ Lower blood pressure
■ Lower cholesterol levels
■ Improved digestion
■ Weight loss
■ Enhanced opportunities for socialization
■ Improved pain control
■ Increased temperature control in response to environmental changes
■ Reduced risk of hypothermia

Despite the many benefits of exercise among older adults, the amount of exercise generally decreases as one ages.

Interventions to promote exercise include helping older adults to choose an exercise program that they enjoy and in which they are motivated to participate. Sample exercise programs include:

■ Walking
■ Aquacise
■ Strength training
■ Yoga

Sleep

The inability to fall asleep and to sleep through the night are among the most frequent complaints of older adults. Many older adults report difficulty falling asleep.

About half of older adults report one or more sleep problems. Key indicators of sleep disorders include:

■ Prolonged periods of difficulty falling asleep or getting back to sleep after night-time awakenings
■ Daytime fatigue or sleepiness

Last name:			First name:		
Sex:	Age:	Weight, kg:	Height, cm:		Date:

Complete the screen by filling in the boxes with the appropriate numbers. Total the numbers for the final screening score.

Screening

A   Has food intake declined over the past 3 months due to loss of appetite, digestive problems, chewing or swallowing difficulties?

0 = severe decrease in food intake
1 = moderate decrease in food intake
2 = no decrease in food intake

B   Weight loss during the past 3 months

0 = weight loss greater than 3 kg (6.6 lbs)
1 = does not know
2 = weight loss between 1 and 3 kg (2.2 and 6.6 lbs)
3 = no weight loss

☐

C   Mobility

0 = bed or chair bound
1 = able to get out of bed / chair but does not go out
2 = goes out

☐

D   Has suffered psychological stress or acute disease in the past 3 months?

0 = yes   2 = no

☐

E   Neuropsychological problems

0 = severe dementia or depression
1 = mild dementia
2 = no psychological problems

☐

F1 Body mass index (BMI) (weight in kg) / (height in m^2)

0 = BMI less than 19
1 = BMI 19 to less than 21
2 = BMI 21 to less than 23
3 = BMI 23 or greater

☐

IF BMI IS NOT AVAILABLE, REPLACE QUESTION F1 WITH QUESTION F2.
DO NOT ANSWER QUESTION F2 IF QUESTION F1 IS ALREADY COMPLETED.

F2 Calf circumference (CC) in cm

0 = CC less than 31
3 = CC 31 or greater

☐

Screening score (max. 14 points)

12–14 points: Normal nutritional status
8–11 points: At risk of malnutrition
0–7 points: Malnourished

☐☐

References
1. Vellas B, Villars H, Abellan G, *et al.* Overview of the MNA® - Its History and Challenges. *J Nutr Health Aging.* 2006;10:456-465.
2. Rubenstein LZ, Harker JO, Salva A, Guigoz Y, Vellas B. Screening for Undernutrition in Geriatric Practice: Developing the Short-Form Mini Nutritional Assessment (MNA-SF). *J. Geront.* 2001; 56A: M366-377
3. Guigoz Y. The Mini-Nutritional Assessment (MNA®) Review of the Literature - What does it tell us? *J Nutr Health Aging.* 2006; 10:466-487.
4. Kaiser MJ, Bauer JM, Ramsch C, et al. Validation of the Mini Nutritional Assessment Short-Form (MNA®-SF): A practical tool for identification of nutritional status. *J Nutr Health Aging.* 2009; 13:782-788.
® Société des Produits Nestlé, S.A., Vevey, Switzerland, Trademark Owners © Nestlé, 1994, Revision 2009. N67200 12/99 10M
For more information: www.mna-elderly.com

FIGURE 5.1   Mini-Nutritional Assessment (MNA).
Source: Nestlé Nutrition Institute.

Sleep patterns are affected by both normal and pathological aging changes. Sleep assessment is the first key to successful sleep management. The Pittsburgh Sleep Quality Index (PSQI; Buysse et al., 1989) is a widely used clinical assessment tool in the form of a self-rated questionnaire, which assesses sleep quality and disturbances over a 1-month time interval. See www.sleep.pitt.edu.

Sleep interventions include the following:

▓ Increase physical activity during the day.

▓ Increase pain medication or alternative pain methods to help older adults suffering from painful conditions to get better rest at night.

▓ Examine the sleep environment. Adjustments in noise and lighting may help older adults to sleep better.

▓ Assess stress levels. Identification and resolution of stressful life factors may help older adults to sleep more peacefully.

▓ Daytime napping may interfere with a good night's sleep. Older adults who choose to nap during the day should limit the duration in order to promote better night-time sleep.

ADULT IMMUNIZATION

One of the greatest advances in primary prevention and public health has been the use of immunizations to prevent disease. Two vaccine-preventable diseases that occur commonly in the elderly with great risk for morbidity and mortality are influenza and viral pneumonia. Influenza results in approximately 42.7 million hospitalizations and deaths annually. Despite this high number and the availability of a preventable vaccine, less than 60% of community-dwelling older adults get vaccinated each year. Vaccination is sometimes contraindicated in people who are allergic to eggs and in those who have experienced a reaction to the vaccine in the past.

Pneumonia can be a serious condition in older adults, and has a higher rate of mortality than in younger people. Pneumonia often has an atypical presentation in older adults. These patients may not experience fever, cough or leukocytosis. They may, however, present with decreased energy, acute onset of confusion, and weight loss.

▓ Estimates indicate that pneumococcal infections are responsible for approximately 100,000 deaths per year.

▓ Pneumonia vaccination is recommended every 10 years or more frequently in high-risk populations.

▓ Many older adults are unvaccinated against pneumonia.

▓ The pneumonia vaccine is effective in preventing 56% to 81% of viral infections.

▓ The pneumonia vaccine is estimated to prevent 80% of pneumonia-related deaths.

■ The vaccine is not useful in some immunocompromised patients.

■ Indications for the pneumonia vaccine:

- Everyone older than 65 years

- People ages 2 to 64 who have chronic illness or live in high-risk areas

- Older adults with chronic lung, heart, kidney, sickle cell disease, or diabetes

ALTERNATIVE AND COMPLEMENTARY HEALTH CARE

The use of herbal medications to treat commonly occurring normal and pathological changes of aging has grown considerably over the past decade. More than a third of older adults have used complementary and alternative medicine in the past 12 months (Barnes, Bloom, & Nahin, 2008). It is important to note that less than half of older adults disclosed the use of alternative medicines with their health care providers.

Complementary and alternative medications are most commonly in Asian cultures (Arcury et al., 2006). The availability of these herbals, often referred to as nutraceuticals, and the anecdotal evidence of their effectiveness have spawned the sudden growth in sales of these supplements. Nutraceuticals also tend to be less expensive than prescription drugs.

Arcury et al. (2006) reported that the use of adjuvant supplements is commonplace in older adults.

Herbal supplements commonly used by older adults include:

■ Vitamins C, D, and E, which have shown some evidence of reducing symptoms of osteoarthritis; however, vitamin E has been shown to result in increased risk of bleeding disorders

■ Black licorice, which has been thought to reduce joint inflammation thereby reducing symptoms of arthritis, may cause irregular heart rhythms and may interact with some diuretics and may lower potassium levels

■ Ginkgo biloba, which is sometimes used by older adults to enhance memory, but there is no evidence to support its effectiveness. It has been shown to increase the risk of bleeding disorders, particularly in patients on other blood thinners

■ Saw palmetto is used by many older men to reduce symptoms of enlarged prostate glands and to prevent prostate cancer; however, it has been shown to be ineffective for this purpose

■ Ginseng is used by older adults to increase energy levels

■ St. John's wort is often used as an alternative or adjunct treatment for mild to moderate depression.

A summary of commonly used herbal medications and their indications is provided in Table 5.2.

TABLE 5.2   Herbal Components Under Study by the National Toxicology Program

---

Aloe vera	Widely used herb, both as a dietary supplement and component of cosmetics. The gel has been used for centuries as a treatment for minor burns and is increasingly being used in products for internal consumption.
Black cohosh	Used to treat symptoms of premenstrual syndrome, dysmenorrhea, and menopause. There is mixed evidence on its effectiveness.
Bladderwrack	A source of iodide used in treatment of thyroid diseases and also used as a component of weight-loss preparations.
Comfrey	Herb consumed in teas and as fresh leaves for salads; however, it contains pyrrolizidine alkaloids, which are known to be toxic. Used externally as an anti-inflammatory agent in the treatment of bruises, sprains, and back pain.
Echinacea purpurea extract	Used as an immunostimulant to treat colds, sore throat, and flu.
Ginkgo biloba extract	Ginkgo biloba is often used to enhance memory, but research has demonstrated that it has no effect on memory.
Ginseng and ginsenosides	Ginsenosides are thought to be the active ingredients in ginseng. Ginseng has been used as a treatment for a variety of conditions, including hypertension, diabetes, and depression, and been associated with various adverse health effects.
Goldenseal	Traditionally used to treat wounds, digestive problems, and infections. Currently used as a laxative, tonic, and diuretic. Mistakenly thought to disguise the presence of other drugs in drug tests.
Green tea extract	Used for its antioxidative properties.
Kava-kava	Kava-kava has psychoactive properties and is sold as a calmative and antidepressant. A recent report of severe liver toxicity has led to restrictions of its sale in Europe and has apparently affected sales in the United States. Some components may alter efficacy/toxicity of therapeutic agents.
Milk thistle extract	Used to treat several liver conditions.
Pulegone	A major terpenoid constituent of the herb pennyroyal, pulegone is found in lesser concentrations in other mints. Pennyroyal has been used as a carminative insect repellent, emmenagogue, and abortifacient. Pulegone has well-recognized toxicity to the liver, kidney, and central nervous system.
Senna	Laxative increasingly used due to the removal of one of the widely used chemical-stimulant-type laxatives from the market. Study in p53+/– transgenic mice is in progress.
Thujone	Terpenoid found in a variety of herbs, including sage and tansy, and in high concentrations in wormwood. Suspected as the causative toxic agent associated with drinking absinthe, a liqueur flavored with wormwood extract.

From the National Toxicology Program (2008).

REFERENCES

Agency for Healthcare Research and Quality. (2014). *Guide to clinical preventive services: Recommendations of the U.S. Preventive Services Task Force.* Rockville, MD: Author. Available from http://www.ahrq.gov/professionals/clinicians-providers/guidelines-recommendations/guide/index.html

Arcury, T. A., Suerken, C. K., Grzywacz, J. G., Bell, R. A., Lang, W., & Quandt, S. A. (2006). Complementary and alternative medicine use among older adults: Ethnic variation. *Ethnicity and Disease, 16*(3), 723–731.

Barnes, P. M., Bloom, B., & Nahin, R. (2008). *Complementary and alternative medicine use among adults and children: United States, 2007* (CDC National Health Statistics Reports #12).

Buysse, D. J., Reynolds III C. F., Monk, T. H., Berman, S. R., & Kupfer, D. J. (1989). The Pittsburgh Sleep Quality Index: A new instrument for psychiatric practice and research. *Journal of Psychiatric Research, 28*(2), 193–213.

Centers for Disease Control and Prevention. (2013). *The state of aging and health in America.* Atlanta, GA: Author. Retrieved from http://www.cdc.gov/features/agingandhealth/state_of_aging_and_health_in_america_2013.pdf

Guigoz, Y. (2006). The Mini-Nutritional assessment (MNA®) review of the literature: What does it tell us? *Journal of Nutritional Health and Aging, 10,* 466–487.

National Toxicology Program. (2008). *Medicinal herbs.* Retrieved from http://ntp.niehs.nih.gov/files/herbalfacts06.pdf

Rubenstein, L. Z., Harker, J. O., Salva, A., Guigoz, Y., & Vellas, B. (2001). Screening for undernutrition in geriatric practice: Developing the short-form mini nutritional assessment (MNA-SF). *Journal of Gerontology, 56A,* M366-M377.

Vellas, B.1., Villars, H., Abellan, G., Soto, M. E., Rolland, Y., Guigoz, Y., ... Garry, P. (2006). Overview of the MNA®: Its history and challenges. *Journal of Nutritional Health and Aging, 10,* 456–465.

6

Environments of Care

SAFETY AND SECURITY ISSUES

Falls

Approximately one third of older adults living at home and up to two thirds of older adults in long-term care facilities fall each year. Falls are a leading cause of injury and death in older adults. About one in seven falls will result in fracture. In patients who are 75 or older, a fall combined with hip fracture is associated with high levels of mortality. Approximately 70% of all fall-related deaths occur in this population of older adults.

The Centers for Disease Control and Prevention shows that fall-related deaths among older adults have increased sharply. Older men tend to die from falls; older women experience more hospitalizations for fall-related hip fracture. Normal changes of aging that can contribute to falls include:

- Sensory alterations: Older adults experience alterations in kinesthetic perception resulting in increased difficulty understanding how their body is moving in space.
- Slowness in the ability to accommodate to changing light conditions, may make it difficult to see uneven ground when moving from light to dark and dark to light.
- Decline in muscular strength may make it difficult for older adults to use their muscular strength to catch themselves once a fall has started.
- Increased curvature in the spine can put the body in an off-center forward-leaning position.

Pathological aging changes also contribute to falls, including:

- Disorders of movement such as Parkinson's disease
- History of stroke, which can weaken one side of the body

■ Sensory impairments like diabetic neuropathy, which can make it difficult to sense the ground underneath the feet.

■ Visual changes like macular degeneration, cataracts, or glaucoma

The highest risk factor for an older adult having a fall is a history of a previous fall. Other factors that increase risk include:

■ Hospitalization within the past 12 months

■ Use of sedatives, hypnotics, psychotropics, diuretics, and antihypertensive medications

■ Poor nutrition and hydration

Fall prevention is critical to avoiding the negative consequences of falling among older adults. Fall prevention begins with assessment.

Prevention strategies include:

■ Removal of fall hazards such as area rugs, exposed electrical cords, and clutter

■ Use of appropriate lighting, especially at night and on stairwells

■ Use of wall-to-wall carpeting or nonskid flooring

■ Exercise interventions to improve balance, strength, and coordination

■ Installation of shower/toilet grab bars

■ Raised toilet seats

■ Use of properly fitted footwear

■ Movement of frequently used items to lower, easily accessible shelves

For further information on risk assessment and prevention of falls in the elderly, refer to the Upright Fall Prevention program website (http://uprightfallprevention.com).

Use of Restraints

Despite the high risk and negative consequences of falls among older adults, restraints are not a reasonable fall-prevention intervention. Restraints do not prevent falls and can increase the risk of injury. A *physical restraint* is defined as a device or object attached or adjacent to a person's body that cannot be removed easily and restricts freedom of movement. Several types of restraints exist.

■ Physical restraints
  • Side rails on hospital beds
  • Vests

- Waist belts and seat belts
- Wrist restraints and "mittens"

■ Chemical restraints

- Sedatives
- Hypnotics

Evidence about the negative effects of the use of restraints is so disturbing that the mandate for restraint-free care can no longer be ignored. Significant morbidity and mortality risk—including asphyxiation and strangulation—is associated with the use of physical restraints, especially when patients are:

■ Confused

■ Agitated

■ Experiencing a new-onset pressure ulcer

■ Suffering from pneumonia

■ Neurologically impaired

Older adults should only be restrained if they are in immediate, physical danger or are hurting themselves or others and then for only a brief period of time. The Omnibus Budget Reconciliation Act of 1987 attempted to curtail restraint use in long-term care facilities. Since this time, the use of restraints has declined significantly. Restraint alternatives should continue to be used to keep residents safe from falls. Some suggestions for patients who have an elevated fall risk might be:

■ Movement of high-risk patients close to the nursing station

■ Mattress placed on the floor

■ Personal attendants

■ Chair or bed alarms

Relocation

Older adults reside in a variety of care environments:

■ Home

■ Senior housing or older-than-50 communities

■ Nursing homes (also known as skilled nursing facilities [SNFs], or long-term care centers)

■ Assisted living facilities (ALFs)

■ Continuing care retirement communities (CCRCs)

Relocation is a significant life event that may play a role in the development or severity of depression among older adults. Relocation of older adults occurs commonly as a result of:

■ Serious illness

■ Decline in functional status, particularly the development of cognitive impairment and/or incontinence

■ Recent fall or fear of falling

■ Loss of spouse or significant other

■ Inability to drive

■ Changes in economic status caused by retirement or the death of the family provider

Because of the negative consequences of relocation, *aging in place* is emphasized as a concept that refers to remaining in one setting throughout the majority of older adulthood.

Translocation syndrome results from a change in surroundings from a home to a nursing home or ALF and may trigger the onset of delirium. The syndrome may manifest as:

■ Impaired physical health

■ Depression

■ Disruption of established behavior patterns

■ Disruption of social relationships

Movement from one environment to another may cause stress and anxiety. Attempting to ease the transition of patients across care settings is important. Some interventions might include:

■ Letting older adults bring favorite things to their new environment to help them transition more effectively.

■ Empowering older adults as much as possible by allowing them to make decisions and articulate needs and desires is a critical factor in assisting their adjustment from one environment to another.

■ Frequent reorientation and the provision of memory aids to orient patients to time, date, and location.

Translocation syndrome is likely to happen during admission to a nursing home or transfer to acute care from a nursing home environment.

■ Close attention to the transition of an older adult across environments of care is essential to minimize the symptoms of translocation syndrome.

■ Older adults must continually be assessed for alterations in function and cognition and be encouraged to participate in the environment at the highest

- Changes in function, cognition, and affect must be diagnosed immediately and appropriate interventions implemented to ensure as safe a transition as possible.
- Little research is available regarding relocation stress and translocation of older adults.

Transportation

Many older adults continue to drive. As the percentage of older adults living in the United States continues to increase, the number of older drivers will also rise. The risk for injuries, hospitalizations, and death from automobile accidents is increased in the older adult population because of the many normal and pathological changes in the neuromuscular and sensory systems, which are listed in Table 6.1. The number of elderly traffic fatalities is expected to more than triple by the year 2030, exceeding the number of alcohol-related fatalities in 1995 by 35% (Burkhardt, Berger, Creedon, & McGavock, 1998).

The growth in the number of older drivers presents additional problems, because cars, roads, and highways were not developed to accommodate the normal changes of aging that occur in older drivers. A large number of older adults thus are unable to drive safely. Driving presents a significant ethical issue of independence among older adults that should not be taken lightly. Older adults who no longer drive face significant issues with transportation. Older adults need transportation for:

- Health care appointments
- Shopping for food and essentials
- Socialization

Although van services are available in many communities to transport older adults, they are not universally available.

- Car and van services usually require advanced scheduling on a first-come, first-served basis.
- Public transportation, such as buses or subways, may be used by older adults to attend their medical appointments.

TABLE 6.1   Aging Changes That Impact Driving

SYSTEM	AGE-RELATED CHANGE
Sensory	Vision
	■ Decline in visual acuity
	■ Decrease in visual accommodation to light and dark
	■ Decline in peripheral vision
	■ Yellowing of the lens of the eye
	■ Increased sensitivity to glare
	Hearing
	■ Increased prevalence of presbycusis

- Public transportation systems are required to accommodate disabilities among older adults.

- Long walks to bus or subway stations may be barriers to using the public transportation system among the elderly.

- Caregivers, friends, and neighbors can sometimes provide assistance with transportation.

- The barriers presented by transportation to health care facilities often are a barrier to medical treatment.

- Lack of transportation to grocery stores may contribute to malnutrition among older adults.

Maintaining Autonomy and Independence

Most older adults prefer to stay in their own homes rather than move to other care environments; the majority of older adults are able to maintain their independence. Approximately 94% of older adults live in community households, either alone or with a relative. Of the 94% who live in the community, most live alone or with a spouse. Living in the same home environment throughout one's life span has advantages and challenges. Some of the advantages are:

- Autonomy over one's living space

- The ability to retain and strengthen social bonds

- The opportunity to form new connections with parents or grandparents who move into the neighborhood

Some of the challenges of remaining at home are:

- Many homes require costly and difficult repairs and maintenance that some older adults can no longer afford or manage.

- Decline in functional status, vision, and hearing can make living at home unsafe.

- Some older adults may require medical care and assistance with activities of daily living and instrumental activities of daily living, which might require driving a great distance in all weather conditions.

- The need for assistance for personal care, which may be costly, and may not be covered by Medicare and private insurance.

Although they may not always be reimbursable, many health care services are available in the home, including:

- Nursing

- Physical therapy

- Occupational therapy

■ Speech–language pathology

■ Assistance with personal care

■ Social work

If an older adult can no longer live at home, attention should be given to protection of his or her personal space in alternate care settings. Autonomy involves setting boundaries to protect one's personal space. Nurses may help older adults protect their autonomy by:

■ Suggesting they bring personal items to the new space

■ Preventing other staff and residents from invading personal space or crossing boundaries

■ Encouraging time in personal space

■ Assessing the amount of personal space, the comfort with eye contact, and the use of physical gestures, such as hand-shaking, to determine the older adult's comfort with these common social norms

COMMUNITY-BASED SERVICES AND RESOURCES

Generally, older adults are formally assessed by an agency to determine their need for home care services. Medicare uses the OASIS (outcome and assessment information set) to evaluate possible recipients of home care services. OASIS is a set of data elements that form a comprehensive assessment for an adult home care patient and provides the basis for measuring patient outcomes for purposes of outcome-based quality improvement. Other community resources funded through grants distributed through the National Association of Area Agencies on Aging or the federal government include:

■ Employment resources

■ Senior-center programs

■ Senior housing

■ Adult day care services

■ Alternative community-based living facilities

It is estimated that family members provide approximately 80% of the care needed by older adults. Caregiving places a tremendous burden on the caregiver, which may result in:

■ Depression

■ Grief

■ Fatigue

■ Decreased socialization

■ Health problems

Respite care for older adults may be found in a local SNF so that the caregiver may vacation and rest. Other supportive services may help to ease caregiver burden, such as:

- Home health aides
- Homemakers
- Chore services
- Meals On Wheels

Caregivers must be encouraged and supported to take care of themselves and pursue their own interests and activities.

RESIDENTIAL FACILITIES

Several types of residential facilities perform care for older adults.

Skilled Nursing Facilities

SNFs may be private or public and may receive reimbursement from Medicare, Medicaid, and private insurances, or residents may self-pay. Nursing services provided in SNFs may include:

- Medication administration
- Wound care
- Daily assessment
- Meals
- Assistance with activities of daily living
- Physical therapy
- Respiratory therapy
- Speech–language pathology services
- Occupational therapy
- Short-term rehabilitation after surgery or medical illness
- Lifetime residential services

The documentation specific to SNFs is known as the Minimum Data Set (MDS). This is a core set of screening, clinical, and functional status elements, including common definitions and coding categories.

- The MDS is the foundation of the comprehensive assessment for all residents of long-term care facilities certified to participate in Medicare or Medicaid.
- The MDS standardizes communication about resident problems and conditions within facilities, between facilities, and between facilities and outside agencies.

Assisted Living Facilities

ALFs were developed in the 1980s to provide supportive residential housing for the rapidly growing elderly population. ALFs place a greater emphasis on autonomy than do nursing homes. They are appealing housing alternatives for older adults with minor to moderate functional impairments. ALFs generally follow a nonmedical, homelike model, focusing on resident

- Autonomy
- Privacy
- Independence
- Dignity
- Respect

ALFs are often less expensive than SNFs, but the nonmedical model also precludes reimbursement by Medicare. Medicare reimbursement for home care services may be provided by an outside home care agency. Services offered at ALFs vary, and often include:

- 24-hour supervision
- Three meals a day plus snacks in a dining-room setting
- A range of personal, health care, and recreational services

Services may be included in the monthly rate, or they may be offered at additional costs. Health care and nursing services available at ALFs vary widely throughout the country. Some facilities have adequate 24-hour coverage, whereas others do not have registered nurses on site. Disparities in state regulations have led to varied interpretations of what ALFs are and what they can do.

Continuing Care Retirement Communities

CCRCs are defined as communities that offer multiple modes of housing incorporating different levels of care (CMS, 2013). They are a housing alternative for older adults that arose in the 1980s with the purpose of facilitating aging in place. CCRCs provide several levels of care, including:

- Independent living
- Assisted living
- Skilled nursing care

Older adults may remain in the CCRC by changing the level of care they receive as changes occur in their health or in their functional or cognitive status. CCRCs are very expensive and require an entrance fee and a monthly payment. However,

- Skilled levels of care are reimbursable under Medicare.
- Independent and assisted living are privately paid.
- Periodic home care services may be reimbursable under Medicare by home care nurses.

Residence in a CCRC requires a commitment to a long-term contract that specifies the housing, services, and nursing care provided. AARP (2007) reports that there are three types of CCRC contracts.

- Extensive contracts include unlimited long-term nursing care at minimal or no increase in monthly fee.
- Modified contracts include a specified amount of long-term care. If chronic conditions require more care beyond the specified time, the older adult is responsible for payments.
- With fee-for-service contracts, the older adult pays the full daily rates for long-term nursing care.

CCRCs originated with religious or social groups interested in caring for members of their communities. More recently, private investors have begun to purchase and operate these communities. Services provided depend on the level of care and range from basic recreational services in independent living to full care and meals in a skilled nursing environment.

HOMELESS ELDERS

Homelessness is a significant problem among the older adult population. Little is known about the homeless older population because these individuals rarely seek health services and, therefore, are difficult to access. The few available studies estimate that there are between 60,000 and 400,000 older homeless adults in the United States. The typical older homeless person is a man. Despite the lack of health services among older homeless adults, this population suffers from:

- Substantial physical disease
- Mental illness
- Alcohol abuse
- Drug abuse

These risk factors increase the prevalence of the following conditions among homeless older adults.

- Morbidity
- Mortality
- Decreased bone density
- Malnutrition
- Hip fracture from falls
- Motor vehicle accidents

REFERENCES

AARP. (2007). *Continuing care retirement communities.* Retrieved from http://www.aarp.org/families/housing_choices/other_options/a2004-02-26-retirementcommunity.html

Burkhardt, J. E., Berger, A. M., Creedon, M., & McGavock, A. T. (1998). *Mobility and independence: Changes and challenges for older drivers.* Washington, DC: Department of Health and Human Services (DHHS), under the auspices of the Joint DHHS/DOT Coordinating Council on Access and Mobility.

Centers for Medicare and Medicaid Services. (2013). *Your guide to choosing a nursing home or other long-term care.* Baltimore, MD: U.S. Department of Health and Human Services. Retrieved from https://www.medicare.gov/Pubs/pdf/02174.pdf

7

Spirituality and Death and Dying

The many aspects of end-of-life nursing care include:

- Communication
- Physical care
- Spiritual care
- Emotional care
- Psychological care
- Assistance with family grieving

PRINCIPLES OF EFFECTIVE END-OF-LIFE CARE

The goal of end-of-life nursing care is to help patients experience a "good death." Palliative care is aimed at providing essential elements to ensure a good death. The World Health Organization (2015) defines palliative care as "an approach that improves the quality of life of patients and their families facing the problem associated with life-threatening illness, through the prevention and relief of suffering by means of early identification and impeccable assessment and treatment of pain and other problems, physical, psychosocial, and spiritual."

The four dimensions of end-of-life care are physical, psychological, social, and spiritual.

Physical Dimension

The physical dimension of end-of-life care ensures that patients are pain free—no older adult should ever die in pain. Caregivers should follow these guidelines:

- Assess regularly for the presence of pain. At the end of life, nonverbal patients should be assessed with pain measurements, such as the PAINAD. Nurses should be proactive in seeking as-needed orders to be able to rapidly

■ Treat with pharmacological and nonpharmacological interventions on a regular schedule (not as needed) to ensure the patient is pain free.

■ Support older adults in maintaining their independence as long as possible.

■ Assistance may be needed when the older adult is no longer able to complete activities of daily living independently.

Other physical symptoms common at the end of life include dyspnea, cough, anorexia, constipation, diarrhea, nausea, vomiting, and fatigue. These symptoms are summarized in Table 7.1.

TABLE 7.1 Physical Symptoms at the End of Life

PHYSICAL SYMPTOM	NURSING INTERVENTIONS
Dyspnea	■ Assess respiratory rate and effort as well as pattern of dyspnea and triggering and relieving factors (i.e., activity). ■ Respiratory rates of more than 20 breaths per minute, labored respirations, use of accessory muscles, and diminished or adventitious lung sounds require follow-up and possible intervention. ■ Administer morphine solution orally or sublingually every 2 hours, as needed. Diuretics (e.g., Lasix), bronchodilators, steroids, antibiotics, anticholinergics, and sedatives should also be considered to ease the sensation of dyspnea and to reduce anxiety. ■ Administer humidified oxygen, as appropriate, to relieve symptoms, especially in those who do not respond to morphine. ■ Keep environment cool and position client for full chest expansion. Many patients who are short of breath prefer to sit upright.
Cough	■ Assess etiology of cough. ■ If from excess fluids, treat accordingly with diuretics (e.g., Lasix). ■ Elevate head of bed. ■ Many patients at the end of life have dryness in their mouths and throats. Ensure proper fluid administration. ■ Administer cough suppressants/depressants, opiates, bronchodilators, and local anesthetics.
Anorexia	■ Lack of appetite is normal at the end of life. Food and fluids at the end of life may create distress and, thus, anorexia does not necessarily need to be treated. Patients who are hungry at the end of life should be provided with comforting foods that bring them pleasure. There should be no dietary restrictions at the end of life. ■ Good oral hygiene, using a soft toothbrush or spongy oral swab, is essential to prevent dryness, mouth sores, dental problems, and infections.
Constipation	■ Recognize the impact of morphine preparations on constipation among older adults and administer prophylactic treatment for constipation. ■ Assess client's self-report as well as physical symptoms of constipation, such as bowel distension, nausea, vomiting, or rectal impaction. ■ Recommended medications include stool softeners such as docusate sodium (Colace) and stimulant laxatives such as senna (Senokot S). ■ Bowel suppositories and enemas may also be used to relieve constipation. ■ Be alert for the progression of constipation to bowel obstruction. This may present as steady abdominal pain and is a medical emergency.

(continued)

TABLE 7.1 Physical Symptoms at the End of Life (*continued*)

PHYSICAL SYMPTOM	NURSING INTERVENTIONS
Diarrhea	■ Assess presence and etiology of diarrhea and treat the cause, if possible. Treating the cause of diarrhea, is important to maintain patient comfort. ■ Ensure adequate fiber and bulk in diet and adequate intake of fluids. ■ Consider the administration of diphenoxylate (Lomotil) or loperamide (Imodium).
Nausea and vomiting	■ Understand that fluctuations in levels of circulating opiate can result in nausea. Maintain stable opiate levels with around-the-clock dosing. ■ Assess client's self-report of nausea, along with aggravating and relieving factors. The use of a diary may be helpful. ■ Assess vomiting as well as aggravating and relieving factors. It is important to note that retching and gagging may occur even in unresponsive clients. ■ Administer antiemetics around the clock (not as needed). Antiemetics that may be effective include prochlorperazine (Compazine) and metoclopramide (Reglan) administered as a rectal suppository, intravenously, or parenterally. ■ Consider the combination preparation of lorazepam (Ativan), diphenhydramine (Benadryl), haloperidol (Haldol), and metoclopramide (Reglan) if antiemetics alone are not effective at relieving symptoms.
Fatigue	■ Fatigue must be recognized as a major source of distress among older adults at the end of life and has a great impact on quality of life. ■ Treatment of symptoms, such as pain, nausea, vomiting, and dyspnea, significantly impact fatigue. ■ Light exercise and activity alternating with periods of rest and relaxation are effective at relieving fatigue. ■ Music and guided imagery may also be helpful for inducing rest and providing stimulation during fatigued periods

Adapted from Matzo and Sherman (2014).

Psychological Dimension

The psychological dimension of end-of-life care focuses on how older adults feel about themselves and their relationships with others. Are there unresolved personal issues? Are there unfinished tasks that need to be completed so that the older adult can feel at ease at the end of life?

■ The end of life provides an opportunity to complete important developmental tasks of aging.

■ Discussing issues with older adults who are approaching the end of life will help to identify uncompleted tasks.

■ Although it may seem too late, some older adults have:

• Completed academic degrees

• Contacted estranged family members

• Been married on their death beds

• Made peace with estranged friends and family members

- Disclosed important aspects of their life histories to children and grandchildren
▦ The nurse may be the one to make the phone call or mediate the discussion between two people who have not spoken in years.
▦ Nurses can play an important role in helping older adults to complete these developmental tasks and experience a good death.
▦ The end of life often involves the development of depression, anxiety, confusion, agitation, and delirium. These symptoms and suggested nursing interventions are described in Table 7.2.

TABLE 7.2   Psychological Symptoms at the End of Life

PSYCHOLOGICAL SYMPTOM	NURSING INTERVENTIONS
Depression	▦ Assess cause of depression; consider unrelieved pain and anticipatory grieving. ▦ Openly discuss older adult's fears and concerns regarding end of life to assist in the resolution of depression. ▦ Refer for counseling. ▦ Implement suicide precautions, if necessary. ▦ Consider administration of antidepressants, including selective serotonin reuptake inhibitors: fluoxetine (Prozac), paroxetine (Paxil), and sertraline (Zoloft); tricyclic antidepressants: amitriptyline (Elavil), imipramine (Tofranil), and nortriptyline (Pamelor); monoamine oxidase inhibitors: phenelzine (Nardil) and tranylcypromine (Parnate); and the other atypical antidepressants (Desyrel) and bupropion (Wellburtin). Although many drugs and drug classes should be discontinued at the end of life, antidepressants should continue to be administered.
Anxiety and agitation	▦ Assess cause of anxiety and agitation; consider unrelieved pain, urinary retention, constipation, and nausea as sources and treat appropriately. ▦ Openly discuss older adults' fears and concerns regarding end of life to assist in the resolution of anxiety-producing issues. ▦ Administer anxiolytics such as lorazepam (Ativan), diazepam (Valium), or clonazepam (Klonopin). However, remember that these medications may result in delirium among older adults. ▦ If anxiolytic medications fail to relieve anxiety, consider the use of barbiturates such as phenobarbital or neuroleptics such as haloperidol (Haldol).
Delirium and acute confusion	▦ Assess delirium using a standardized instrument, such as a confusion assessment method (CAM). ▦ Delirium is a frequent occurrence at end of life as a result of life-threatening conditions and treatment strategies. ▦ Immediate detection and removal of the cause of delirium will enhance the patient's recovery to the quickest extent possible. ▦ While the delirium is resolving, it is important to keep the older adult safe through the use of detection systems to alert caregivers of wandering behavior and implementing fall-prevention strategies. ▦ A calm, soft-spoken approach to care is necessary, and the older adult with delirium should not be forced to participate in caregiving activities that cause anxiety or agitation.

Social Dimension

The social dimension of end-of-life care identifies roles that older adults have occupied and determines whether they have disengaged from these roles. With the rising number of older adults caring for grandchildren, an aging grandmother may be concerned about who will care for her grandchildren when she passes away.

■ Older adults may be employed and worry about how their job responsibilities will be met upon their death.

■ Older adults may be caregivers to ill or cognitively impaired spouses or siblings, and the loved one's future care is likely to be a concern.

Spiritual Dimension

The spiritual dimension of end-of-life care allows the older adult to transcend from this life into another existence.

■ If the older adult has explored the meaning of his or her life and has an expectation of an afterlife, death may be peaceful.

■ Older adults often continue to struggle with the meaning of life even at the end.

■ The presence of spirituality in the lives of older adults once was not acknowledged.

■ The original work of Rowe and Kahn (1997) on successful aging neglected to include the component of spirituality.

■ More recently, spirituality has been identified as an integral component of health and functioning.

■ Spirituality provides a framework within which people conduct the search for meaning and purpose in life.

■ Spirituality differs from religion, which specifically concerns the spiritual beliefs and practices held by organized groups (e.g., Buddhist, Catholic, Protestant, Jewish).

■ Religion is defined by Koenig et al. (2001) as "an organized system of beliefs, practices, rituals and symbols designed

a. to facilitate closeness to the sacred or transcendent (God, higher power, or ultimate truth/reality)

b. to foster an understanding of one's relation and responsibility to others living together in a community" (Koenig et al., 2001, p. 18)

■ Although many people pursue spirituality through a specific religion, participation in organized religion is not a prerequisite for spiritual activity at the end of life.

■ Many older adults do not affiliate with an organized religion, yet possess a

■ It is of great importance that nurses understand that spirituality and the practice of religion vary greatly among older adults.

■ The presence of spirituality has been associated with relief from physical, mental, and addictive disorders and with enhanced quality of life and survival.

■ The influence of spirituality on the health and functioning of older adults as well as a good death indicates the need to plan care that incorporates spiritual needs.

■ Older adults who engage in religious and spiritual practice often cope better psychologically and have better physical health than those who don't (Koenig, 2007).

■ The presence of spirituality has been associated with relief from physical, mental, and addictive disorders and enhanced quality of life and survival.

■ Understanding the role of spirituality in death is the first step toward spiritual care for older adults.

■ Spiritual care for older adults begins with an assessment of:

- The individual's beliefs and practices
- What spirituality means to the client
- Whether the client is affiliated with a specific religion and is actively involved
- Whether spirituality is a source of support and strength
- Whether the client has any special religious traditions, rituals, or practices he or she likes to follow

■ Many spiritual assessment scales are available, including Stoll's Spiritual Assessment Guide and O'Brien's Spiritual Assessment Scale. These instruments may be helpful in conducting spiritual assessments of older adults.

■ From the spiritual assessment, deficits in the older adult's spiritual needs may be found and interventions implemented to help the older adult improve his or her spiritual connectedness.

■ Nurses should encourage religious and spiritual beliefs and practices in all environments of care, as allowed by institutional policy.

■ It is important for nurses to be aware of the availability of religious personnel within each facility and call on these members of the interdisciplinary team to help older adults whenever necessary.

■ Spiritual counseling and praying with the patient can be great sources of comfort to the patient and his or her family.

- A hallmark of palliative care is communication among caregivers, families, and patients.
- Nurses can play an instrumental role in bringing together interdisciplinary teams to plan care for dying older adults.

- Team conferences should be held regularly to plan care and to assess effectiveness in meeting patients' multidimensional palliative care needs.
  - It is important that both the patient and family are encouraged to participate in care planning and evaluation.
- Different cultures view death differently.

ADVANCE DIRECTIVES

Advance directives allow older adults to participate in and direct health care decisions at the end of life or in the event that they are unable to do so at some time in the future. Advance directives include the right to accept or refuse medical or surgical treatment.

- In 1990, the Patient Self-Determination Act was created to require every health care institution to maintain specific policies and procedures regarding advance directives for every adult who receives health care in that institution.
- Every older adult has the right to prepare advance directives and be informed of the provider's policies that govern the utilization of these rights.
- Failure to comply with the act may result in the facility's loss of Medicare and Medicaid payments.
- Advance directives provide a way for older adults to make decisions about their lives and health care prior to becoming ill. Although it is not required that older adults make these decisions (and many do not), it is required that hospitals provide clients with the option to do so.
- The use of verbal statements, living wills, and durable powers of attorney are all considered legitimate advance directives for future health care treatment decisions.
- Older adults may be encouraged to complete advance directives in order to have their wishes followed at the end of life.
- Nurses have a unique opportunity to encourage the development of advance directives in all environments of care.
- Families' decisions about continuing or removing life-sustaining treatments may conflict with health care providers' recommendations. In these cases, it is most appropriate to determine the client's wishes.
- Cultural values influence the decision to sustain or withhold nutrition and hydration at the end of life.
- Verbal statements regarding potential health care problems and possible treatment decisions may be made by older adults to health care providers and trusted friends and family.

▦ Verbal statements indicate a thoughtful approach to decisions that are consistent with ethical principles and with the older adult's past decisions. They may be used to make health care decisions when the older adult is no longer able to do so.

▦ If verbal statements are spoken to health care providers, documenting them in the patient record provides the best evidence of the patient's wishes.

▦ Living wills are a written statement about preferences for life-sustaining treatment.

▦ Living wills provide older adults with the opportunity to describe any life-sustaining treatment they wish to accept or reject should they experience a terminal condition or a permanent state of unconsciousness and are not able to participate in health care treatment decisions.

▦ Because living wills are written forms generally filed with the older adult's medical record, their usefulness is dependent on the health care provider's ability to implement the older adult's wishes.

▦ Similar to a power of attorney for financial decisions, older adults may designate a trusted person to make health care decisions on their behalf.

▦ Durable power of attorney for health care or medical power of attorney extends the power to make health care decisions in the event that the decision-making capacity of the older adult is impaired.

▦ A durable power of attorney may receive diagnostic information, analyze potential treatment options, act as an advocate for the client, and consent to or refuse care.

▦ A durable power of attorney is a legal advance directive that offers greater flexibility than a living will. The document is not limited to life-sustaining measures; it may apply to nursing home placement, surgery, or other forms of nonemergency treatment.

▦ The greatest limitation of the durable power of attorney is the requirement of having a person who is willing to serve in the role of substitute decision maker.

▦ If older adults have outlived all their significant others and do not have anyone to serve as a surrogate decision maker, they may petition for or hire a court-appointed power of attorney in order to benefit from the flexibility offered by a durable power of attorney for health care.

▦ A will is a written document that provides for the distribution of financial assets upon a person's death.

▦ Wills are important documents to help older adults determine the disposition of their assets, but they do not generally provide advance direction regarding health care decisions.

▦ Do not resuscitate (DNR) orders are direct orders from health providers to forego cardiopulmonary resuscitation in the event of cardiopulmonary arrest. In addition to a DNR, a patient may have a declaration about life-prolonging procedures that details patient preferences regarding the use of

HOSPICE AND PALLIATIVE CARE

Hospice care at the end of life is an extremely valuable yet underused, resource. Although hospices have provided compassionate palliative care for terminally ill persons and their families in the United States for more than 20 years, many people are still not aware of these services.

■ The greatest growth in hospice use over the past decade is among older clients (Hospice Association of America, 2007).

■ Hospice is a philosophy of care for dying persons and their families that affirms life and empowers dying persons to live with dignity, encouraging them to remain alert and pain free.

■ It involves families and loved ones in giving care that emphasizes quality of life.

■ The hospice team facilitates the establishment of an environment in which dying persons and their families have satisfactory psychological and spiritual preparation for death.

■ The hospice philosophy supports the belief that dying is a natural extension of the living process.

■ The traditional goals of hospice care are to:
  • Relieve the pain and suffering of the terminally ill
  • Make a good death possible
  • Help the family
  • Assist in the search for the meaning of life and death

GRIEVING

Nurses' work with older adults at the end of life does not end when the older client passes away. Sadness is a common symptom of the normal mourning process. Nurses can help families through the grieving process. Grieving begins before the older adult dies and proceeds differently for each family.

Types of grief include acute, anticipatory, and dysfunctional.

■ Acute grief occurs in response to feelings of loss.

■ Anticipatory grief occurs in anticipation of an impending loss.

■ Dysfunctional or complicated grief occurs when the duration of symptomatology is prolonged, resulting in impaired psychosocial functioning.

Kübler-Ross (1964) describes several stages of grieving that must be experienced for successful resolution of the loss. Progress through these stages is unpredictable, but necessary.

■ Denial (this isn't happening to me)

- Bargaining (I promise I'll be a better person if …)
- Depression (I don't care anymore)
- Acceptance (I'm ready for whatever comes)

Families who have lost an older relative never just "get over it." Signs that a grieving person is in distress may include:

- Weight loss
- Substance abuse
- Depression
- Prolonged difficulty with sleep
- Physical problems
- Suicidal ideation
- Lack of personal hygiene

A grief assessment helps to determine the type of grief, a family's reactions, the stages and tasks to be completed, and additional factors influencing the grief process.

- Once the nurse gathers information on the family's grief, an active listening approach assists with resolution.
- Utilizing principles of therapeutic communication, nurses identify problems with the grieving process and allow the family to talk through the situation, sharing experiences as appropriate so that the family members know they are not alone.
- Nurses may identify support systems, such as bereavement specialists and support groups.
- The nurse should encourage the family to conduct activities and attend rituals surrounding the older adult's death, even if this is difficult, because these ceremonies provide closure to the older adult's life.
- Individuals may need a referral for professional assistance to accomplish grieving effectively.
- It is important to note that grief work is never completely finished, but the pain diminishes over time.

WIDOWHOOD

Several means exist to assist widows and widowers through the intensive grief period immediately after the loss of a spouse, including:

- Support from family and health care professionals
- Widowhood support groups

■ Clergy visitation

■ Social services

■ If the family had hospice services in place prior to the death of the spouse, support services continue for 1 year after the death.

■ After the loss of a spouse, it is especially important for health care professionals to monitor the health status of the recently widowed older adult.

■ It is during this period of intense grief that the widowed spouse may ignore self-care activities, become malnourished, not take medications appropriately, refuse social interactions, or indulge in substance abuse.

■ The loss of intimacy after many years with a partner can seriously impact one's life and health.

■ Physical and psychological closeness to someone is an important part of self-concept and self-esteem; widowhood after a long marriage can greatly impact one's self-image.

■ The loss of a spouse and entrance into widowhood is generally perceived as a serious life event. It is classified as severe social stress that affects the health of the widowed individual.

■ Older widowers tend to have more problems with household management after the loss of their wives, and older widows tend to experience increased financial burdens after the death of their husbands.

REFERENCES

Hospice Association of America. (2007). *Hospice facts and figures.* Retrieved from http://www.nahc.org/HAA/2007HospiceFactsStatistics.pdf

Koenig, H. G. (2007). Religion and remission of depression in medical inpatients with heart failure/pulmonary disease. *Journal of Nervous and Mental Disease, 195*(5), 389–395.

Koenig, H. G., McCullogh, M., & Larson, D. B. (2001). *Handbook of religion and health.* New York, NY: Oxford University Press.

Kübler-Ross, E. (1964). *On death and dying.* New York, NY: Macmillan.

Matzo, M. L., & Sherman, D. W. (Eds.). (2014). *Palliative care nursing: Quality of care to the end of life.* New York, NY: Springer Publishing Company.

Rowe, J. W., & Kahn, R. L. (1997). Successful aging. *Aging, 10,* 142–144.

World Health Organization. (2015). *Definition of palliative care.* Retrieved from http://www.who.int/cancer/palliative/definition/en

8

Acute and Chronic Physical Illnesses

As the older adult population continues to grow and life spans continue to increase, the number of chronic illnesses among older adults will also increase. These chronic conditions require effective disease management. As of 2012, about half of all American adults had at least one chronic condition, about a quarter of adults had two or more chronic conditions (Ward, Schiller, & Goodman, 2014). Many of the conditions discussed in this chapter are the direct result of lifestyle choices. Federal guidelines recommend a minimum of 30 minutes of aerobic activity 5 days per week or approximately 2 ½ hours of physical activity per week. Less than a quarter of adults over 75 meet current guidelines for aerobic activity, and only 12.1% meet guidelines for strength-building activities. In addition to a lack of exercise, 37% of American adults consume less than one serving of fruit daily, and 22.6% consume less than one serving of vegetables per day (Centers for Disease Control and Prevention [CDC], 2013).

CARDIAC AND PERIPHERAL VASCULAR PROBLEMS

Hypertension

Hypertension results from many nonmodifiable and modifiable risk factors and lifestyle behaviors. It is a serious risk factor for the development of many types of cardiovascular and renal diseases. (See Table 4.1 for a list of the JNC-VIII criteria for blood pressure.) The risk of developing hypertension increases with age. Among people 75 and older, approximately 72% of men and 80% of women have hypertension. Hypertension is considered a silent killer because it has no signs and symptoms.

- Approximately 18.5% of people with hypertension are unaware that they have it.
- The American Heart Association (2005) estimates that, of those with hypertension, about 25% are not on medication and many more are on inadequate hypertensive therapy

■ The combination of diabetes and smoking is more dangerous than either risk factor alone, and increases the risk of adverse events resulting from hypertension.

Nursing interventions for the treatment of hypertension include:

■ Dietary modification: A low-salt, low-cholesterol, low-fat diet is preferred. For patients with kidney damage as a result of hypertension, a low-protein diet is also recommended.

- Exercise: Current federal recommendations are for a minimum of 30 minutes per day on most (5) days for a total of 150 minutes per week.
- Stress management
- Weight loss, if indicated
- Smoking cessation, if indicated

■ Medication management: For hypertension, like most of the diseases associated with aging, the preferred first-line treatment is diet and lifestyle modification. In a trial of patients with stage I hypertension, approximately 40% were able to completely avoid the use of medications through the use of diet and lifestyle changes alone. Because of the damaging effects of hypertension across all organ systems, if diet and lifestyle changes alone are ineffective in reducing blood pressure, pharmacological therapy must be initiated.

- First-line pharmacological therapy consists of thiazide diuretics, such as hydrochlorothiazide (HCTZ) or Diuril; and beta blockers, such as atenolol (Tenormin), labetalol (Normodyne), or propranolol (Inderal). Angiotensin-converting enzyme (ACE) inhibitors, such as benazepril (Lotensin) or captopril (Capoten); and calcium channel blockers, such as amlodipine (Norvasc) and diltiazem (Cardizem), are used for first-line therapy only when diuretics and beta blockers are contraindicated.
- Side effects of antihypertensive medications may include dry, persistent cough (ACE inhibitors), and erectile dysfunction.

Congestive Heart Failure

Congestive heart failure (CHF) is a chronic medical condition that results in acute medical crisis; it occurs more often as people age.

■ In the United States, approximately 4.8 million people have CHF, and each year, 400,000 new cases are diagnosed.

■ Approximately one half of older adults with CHF will die within 5 years of being diagnosed with the disease.

■ The presentation and outcome of CHF are often influenced by the presence of co-morbidity.

- About 80% of all clients with CHF are age 65 and older.
- CHF affects approximately one million older adults annually.

- CHF is a multifaceted disease exacerbated by normal changes in the heart that accompany aging.
- CHF commonly occurs when the pumping ability of the heart is impaired and it can no longer deliver adequate blood circulation to supply the body's metabolic requirements.
- CHF may be used to refer to either left ventricular failure or right ventricular failure. The pathology in most older adults is left ventricular dysfunction.
- CHF is often caused by a myocardial infarction (MI) and coronary artery disease.

■ Other causes of CHF include:
- Valvular dysfunction
- Arrhythmias
- Infections
- Rheumatic heart disease
- Hyperthyroidism
- Anemia
- Excess salt and fluid intake
- Steroid administration
- The discontinuation of cardiac medications

■ The typical presentation of CHF in older adults includes the sudden development of:
- Shortness of breath
- Dyspnea with exertion
- Fatigue
- Weakness
- Alteration in function
- Change in cognition
- Pedal edema
- Fluid in lungs

■ Other symptoms may include:
- Diaphoresis
- Tachycardia
- Palpitations
- Anorexia
- Insomnia

■ Normal and pathological aging changes may make the early assessment and treatment of CHF difficult.

- Pedal edema or weight gain due to CHF may be confused with normal pedal edema that occurs with aging or the side effects of steroid treatment for chronic obstructive pulmonary disease (COPD).
- Altered cough reflex may prevent early detection of pulmonary changes.
- Chest pain or tightness, fatigue, general weakness, a nonproductive cough, and insomnia may be commonly attributable to other conditions of aging and orthopnea.

Nurses play an important role in identifying early symptoms of CHF through awareness of common signs and symptoms in older adults. Effective management of CHF in older adults includes:

▓ Education about
- Self-care—alternating periods of activity with rest
- Low-salt or sodium-restricted diets
- Medication administration involving a combination of ACE inhibitors, such as benazepril (Lotensin) or captopril (Capoten); digoxin; and diuretics

▓ Early identification of symptoms
- Administration of diuretics to decrease cardiac workload; without further symptoms, combined with adequate urinary output, older adults may be evaluated for several hours in the emergency department, home, or out-patient facility and then discharged.
- The persistence of symptoms or failure to reduce cardiac output requires further treatment and hospitalization.

Angina and MI

Angina occurs in approximately 13.7% of women and 21% of men aged 65 to 69.

▓ The *Merck Manual of Geriatrics* (Beers & Berkow, 2000) reports that MI occurs in approximately 35% of older adults; 60% of hospitalizations due to acute MI occur in persons 65 years and older.

▓ A variety of factors can precipitate angina and MI among older adults, the most common of which is coronary artery disease.

▓ Other causes of MI include
- Alular dysfunction
- Arrhythmias
- Infections
- Rheumatic heart disease
- Hyperthyroidism
- Anemia
- Excess salt and fluid intake

- Steroid administration
- Discontinuation of cardiac medications

■ Angina results from a lack of oxygen supply to the heart muscle due to reduced blood flow around the heart's blood vessels.

■ Angina is the most common symptom of myocardial ischemia and is experienced commonly among older adults with coronary artery disease.

■ MI is a serious, sudden heart condition usually characterized by varying degrees of chest pain or discomfort, weakness, sweating, nausea, and vomiting, sometimes causing loss of consciousness.

■ MI occurs when a part of the heart muscle dies because of sudden total interruption of blood flow to that area.

■ The classic clinical presentation of MI regardless of gender results in pain. Women are more likely to present with atypical symptoms, such as fatigue, shortness of breath, upper back and upper abdominal pain. In older adults, the pain response may be blunted.

■ The pain and dysrhythmias of MI are often more serious in older adults than in younger clients as a result of both normal and pathological aging changes.

■ Older adults may *not* exhibit the usual signs of MI, such as:
- Crushing, radiating chest pain
- Gray or cyanotic skin
- Diaphoresis
- Severe anxiety
- Nausea and vomiting
- Hiccoughs

■ In older adults, symptoms of MI may be insidious or vague (silent heart attack), because older adults may
- Be reluctant to complain
- Have communication barriers, such as changes in cognition or hearing
- Have poststroke aphasia

■ Some older adults may attribute the symptoms of angina and MI to
- Normal aging changes
- Symptoms of other disease processes

■ Older adults may not have chest pain but may complain about any combination of
- Pain in the back, shoulder, jaw, or abdomen
- Diminished level of consciousness or acute confusion
- Nausea and vomiting
- Hypotension

- Dizziness or syncope
- Transient ischemic attack (TIA)
- Cerebral vascular accident (CVA)
- Weakness
- Fatigue
- Falls
- Restlessness
- Incontinence

Nurses play an important role in identifying early symptoms of angina and MI. Because both of these diseases may present as pain among older adults, attention to pain complaints must be considered seriously and proper assessment implemented.

■ Nurses' beliefs that pain is a natural and expected part of aging is among one of the most prevalent myths that prevent appropriate treatment of angina and MI among older adults.

■ Many older adults tend to hesitate to report pain because they think nothing can be done to manage the pain and/or they are afraid to bother the nurse.

■ Objective pain is aided by the presence of many standardized tools for assessing pain in older adults. A frequently used measure of pain evaluation is a numeric rating scale in which clients are asked to indicate the pain they are experiencing on a scale of 0 to 10, with 0 being no pain and 10 being the worst pain imaginable.

■ After pain complaints are validated, further symptoms of angina and MI should be evaluated with the interdisciplinary team using
- Electrocardiograms
- Cardiac enzyme evaluation

■ MIs are medical emergencies and must be managed accordingly.

■ Drug therapy for chronic angina usually involves:
- Daily application of nitroglycerin patches (Nitrodisc, Nitro-Dur) to enhance perfusion to the cardiac vessels
- Maintenance of sublingual nitroglycerin pills (Nitrostat, Nitrolingual) in the case of angina; proper instruction regarding the application of patches and the administration of sublingual nitroglycerin is needed
- Lipid-lowering medications known popularly as statins, which are often effective in reducing further occlusion of the cardiac vessels
- Assessing cholesterol levels in clients within the normal range in order to reduce morbidity and mortality among this population
- Selective beta blocker medications, such as acebutolol (Sectral) and atenolol (Tenormin), which also may be prescribed to prevent MI in patients with angina

■ Nurses may also implement programs of
  - Weight loss for obese clients
  - Physical activity
  - Low-cholesterol and low-sodium diets

Peripheral Vascular Disease

Peripheral vascular disease (PVD) is a broad term that refers to altered circulation in the extremities—usually the legs—resulting from poor vascularization over many years.

■ Risk factors for PVD include
  - Diabetes
  - Smoking
  - High-fat diets
  - Sedentary lifestyle

■ Intermittent claudication refers to vascular-related pain that develops in the muscles of the legs while walking.
  - Symptoms may be misattributed to arthritis or neuropathy.
  - PVD is assessed by the amount of distance ambulated before the onset of pain.

■ Surgical procedures may be available to improve circulation in the case of disabling PVD.

■ When tolerated, exercise has been found to be effective to promote collateral circulation.

■ Deep vein thrombosis (DVT) occurs when a blood clot, or thrombus, develops in the large veins of the legs; DVT is a major risk of immobility after surgery.
  - DVT is characterized by acute onset of pain and edema in the affected extremity.
  - Because a clot may become free and clog a major artery, such as a pulmonary artery, DVT is a medical emergency and should be treated accordingly with surgery and/or clot-dissolving medications.
  - Patients at high risk may continue to remain on Coumadin and should be counseled to wear antiembolitic stockings.

RESPIRATORY PROBLEMS

Pneumonia

Pneumonia is the leading cause of death from infectious disease in the United States and the overall sixth leading cause of death in the United States (Institute for Clinical Systems Improvement, 2003). The death rate from pneumonia is especially high among older adults who have had surgery or mechanical ventilation.

■ Normal changes of aging, such as lowered immune status, impact pneumonia as do changes in respiratory function, including:

- Altered cough reflex
- Diminished airway clearance

■ Further risk factors for pneumonia are the presence of chronic diseases and conditions such as:

- COPD
- CHF
- Gastroesophageal reflux disease (GERD)
- Impaired swallowing
- Tube feeding
- Impaired mobility
- Alterations in levels of nutrition

■ The traditional symptoms of pneumonia are often absent or difficult to assess among older adults. These symptoms include:

- Cough
- Fever
- Dyspnea
- Purulent sputum
- Pleuritic chest pain

■ Most older adults with pneumonia have a presentation of disease that consists of:

- Anorexia
- Confusion, delirium, or change in behavior
- Altered functional abilities
- Decompensation caused by underlying illnesses

■ Nursing interventions for the treatment of pneumonia include:

- The administration of medications aimed at destroying the causative organism or virus
- Proper diet
- Hydration
- Treatment of fever and discomfort with acetaminophen or nonsteroidal anti-inflammatory drugs (NSAIDs)
- Respiratory therapy, such as postural drainage

- Evaluation of complications that require follow-up or further therapy, including:
  - Dyspnea
  - Worsening cough
  - Onset or worsening of chills
  - Fever occurring more than 48 hours after drug therapy is started
  - Intolerance of the medications

Influenza

- Influenza, commonly known as the flu, is a contagious viral disease that frequently infects the population during the winter months.
- The CDC (2007a) reports that between 10% and 20% of the U.S. population is infected with the flu each year.
- The flu is often only a mild disease in healthy children and adults, manifesting symptoms such as fever, sore throat, dry cough, headache, and aching muscles.
- Older adults are more likely to develop life-threatening complications from the flu, such as:
  - Changes in mental status
  - Dehydration
  - Pneumonia
  - Extreme tiredness
- Each year, approximately 36,000 U.S. residents die from influenza, and 114,000 are hospitalized from the disease (CDC, 2007a).
- Older adults may present with flu symptoms differently than their younger counterparts.
- In older adults, the classic symptoms of cough, congestion, nausea, and vomiting may be absent or attributed to other disease processes.
- Older adults with the flu may present with acute confusion or delirium.
- Nursing interventions include:
  - Nutrition
  - Hydration
  - Rest
- Symptomatic treatment of the disease includes the use of fever reducers, such as acetaminophen or ibuprofen, and cough suppressants.
- Vaccination remains the most commonly used method of preventing and reducing the impact of the flu.

- Vaccination is required each year because the flu viruses change constantly and unpredictably.
- Medicare currently reimburses providers for annual influenza vaccinations.

Tuberculosis

Some characteristics of tuberculosis are:

- Infectious disease caused by *Mycobacterium tuberculosis*
- Spread through droplets
- Infection may be prevented by respiratory clearance mechanisms (50% from high carriers)
- Lodges in lung and results in tubercle
- Long latency period

The epidemiology of tuberculosis is:

- One third of the world's population is infected with latent disease (4%–6% of U.S. residents).
- 8 to 10 million worldwide will develop active infections annually.
- It is primarily a disease of young adults, but the risk of tuberculosis among older adults is significantly increased in the institutionalized population.

Symptoms of tuberculosis include:

- Fatigue
- Anorexia
- Weight loss
- Cough
- Night sweats
- Fever
- Chest pain
- May have peripheral involvement

Diagnosis of tuberculosis:

- Purified protein derivative (PPD) or Mantoux test result of 5 mm or greater
- QuantiFERON-TB (better at detecting latent infection and immunization with bacillus Calmette-Guérin)
- Chest x-ray
- Lab—acid fast bacilli (may take 3–8 weeks)

■ Strong clinical suspicion

■ Multiple-drug treatment regimen with isoniazid, rifampin, pyrazinamide, and ethambutol

Obstructive Airway Disease

Obstructive airway diseases collectively rank as the fourth leading cause of death in the United States. Chronic bronchitis, asthma, and emphysema are the three major obstructive airway diseases that collectively represent COPD, found prevalently among older adults.

■ Chronic bronchitis is caused by the inflammation of respiratory passages and results in edema and the development of sputum that tends to make breathing very difficult and in some cases impossible.

■ Asthma is manifested by the onset of bronchospasm, mucosal edema, and large amounts of sputum production.

■ Asthma is on the rise in the United States; the incidence and death rates of the disease are increasing among all age groups, including older adults.

■ Some older adults grow old with the disease and some experience new-onset asthma in their later years.

■ Emphysema results from damage to the alveoli (the functional units in the lungs), which results in a reduction in the lung tissue available for aeration (alveolar-capillary diffusion interface).

■ COPD can be the result of many factors, including:
  • Air pollution
  • Smoking

■ Nursing interventions for COPD vary but the goals of all disease therapies are to:
  • Maintain patent airways with the use of suction and medication.
  • Teach patients about the use of inhalers.
  • Teach patients about energy conservation.
  • Teach safe and effective oxygen administration.
  • Administer steroid medications as needed to decrease airway inflammation.
  • Administer opioids that have been supported as safe and effective in reducing terminal dyspnea and respiratory distress at the end of life.

GASTROINTESTINAL PROBLEMS

Gastroesophageal Reflux Disease

■ GERD occurs frequently in older adults as a result of improper closure of the lower esophageal sphincter.

■ This leads to regurgitation of stomach acid into the esophagus, leading to

■ GERD places older adults at higher risk for esophageal cancers.

■ Risk factors of GERD include (Miller, 2007):

- Diets high in fat, caffeine, chocolate, peppermint, and garlic
- Alcoholism
- Consumption of large meals
- History of hiatal hernia
- Smoking
- Use of the following medications:
  - Calcium channel blockers
  - Nitrates
  - NSAIDs
  - Anticholinergics

■ Signs and symptoms of GERD include:

- Foul taste in mouth
- Heartburn
- Nausea
- Belching
- Dry cough

■ Treatment usually involves:

- Administration of proton pump inhibitors, such as Nexium, Pepcid, or Protonix
- Diet modifications to avoid causative foods
- Elevating the head of the bed
- Smoking cessation

HEMATOLOGICAL PROBLEMS

Anemia

Anemia is a pathological illness among older adults generally resulting from abnormal hemoglobin and hematocrit levels. Older adults with anemia must be assessed to determine the responsible pathology.

■ Medications may cause anemia among older adults.

- Proton pump inhibitors taken for more than 5 years decrease the amount of intrinsic factor available for vitamin B_{12} absorption, resulting in macrocytic anemia.

■ Other risk factors for anemia include

- Crohn's disease

- Gastritis
- Surgical procedures, such as ileostomies or colectomies or small bowel resection
- Cancer
- Renal disease
- HIV
- Other diseases that decrease bone marrow production

■ Assessment for anemia includes frequent evaluation of hemoglobin, hematocrit, and associated blood values specific to the type of anemia.

■ Treatment includes:
  - Diet high in protein and iron
  - Vitamin supplementation

GENITOURINARY PROBLEMS

Urinary Tract Infections

Urinary tract infections are the most common type of infection among older adults and are caused by an accumulation of pathological bacteria in the urine. The rate of urinary tract infections increases significantly among the institutionalized elderly.

■ The symptoms of urinary tract infections are:
  - Incontinence
  - New or increased confusion
  - Falls
  - Urinary frequency
  - Dysuria
  - Suprapubic discomfort
  - Fever
  - Costovertebral tenderness

■ Diagnosis generally involves the collection of a urine specimen for culture and sensitivity.

■ Antibiotic treatment should occur only in the presence of symptoms.
  - A short course of antibiotics is usually recommended. Prolonged treatment may result in vaginitis in older women.
  - Treatment for longer periods of time may be needed among the older population due to their decreased natural immune responses.

■ In-dwelling catheters should be avoided when possible due to the increased risk of developing infections.

SEXUALLY TRANSMITTED DISEASES

Although health care providers are becoming increasingly knowledgeable regarding the unique needs of older adults, the sexuality of this population remains largely unrecognized. Nurses often ignore the sexuality of older adults during assessments, assuming that this aspect of human functioning is no longer applicable. The possibility of an older adult contracting a sexually transmitted disease (STD) is real; these diseases include:

■ *Neisseria gonorrhoreae* (gonorrhea)
  • May be asymptomatic in women but painful in men
  • Screen with smear
  • Treatment:
    – Ceftriaxone
    – Ciprofloxacin
    – Levofloxacin

■ *Treponema palladium* (syphilis)
  • May be asymptomatic in both men and women but they both may be carriers
  • Can result in late cardiovascular and neurological effects
  • Screening is complicated
  • Should test exposed individuals
  • Treatment includes antibiotics such as penicillin

■ *Chlamydia trachomatis* (chlamydia)
  • More than 15 strands of this virus
  • The most common STD
  • Major risk factor for pelvic inflammatory disorder
  • May be asymptomatic in women but painful in men
  • Assessment includes a screen with smear (clean cervical os)
  • Treatment:
    – Azithromycin or doxycycline or ceftriaxone

■ Herpes types 1 and 2
  • Genital herpes
  • One in five individuals has herpes
  • Spread through direct contact with lesions during sexual encounters
  • Screen for morphology of lesions

- Treatment:
  - Acyclovir
  - Famciclovir
  - Valacyclovir (first episode, recurrence, and suppression regimens)
- Human papillomavirus
  - Group of more than 70 viruses that affect genital mucous membranes
  - May be asymptomatic
  - May be associated with some cancers
- Nurses must conduct sexual assessments on older adults with the same frequency as other system assessments. Lack of experience and general discomfort with sexuality among health care providers are often barriers to assessing and managing the sexuality needs of older adults.
- The PLISSIT (permissions, limited information, specific suggestions, and intensive therapy) Model of Sex Therapy (Annon, 1976) guides sexual assessment and intervention of older adults; it has been widely used among younger populations. It suggests that one should ask for permission to discuss sexual issues, give information and suggestions for sexual intercourse, and give therapy surrounding the concept of sexuality.
- The assessment of older adults' sexuality should take place in a quiet area that affords clients necessary privacy.
- The establishment of a trusting relationship between the health care provider and client is essential.
- Nurses must be cautious to be respectful of older adults' sexual beliefs and practices and must prevent judgmental thoughts and comments.
- Appropriate history information regarding sexuality include:
  - Number and history of partners
  - Sexual practices
  - Physical signs and symptoms of sexual problems
  - Presence of problems
  - Level of satisfaction with current sexuality
  - Use of protection and precautions; in the older adult population, STDs such as syphilis, genital herpes, and hepatitis may remain from earlier years and be passed unknowingly to partners.

CANCER

- Although the presence of cancer is seen in all populations, the incidence and prevalence of cancer is disproportionate in the elderly population.
- Approximately 75% of all malignancies in the United States occur among older adults, who, at present, constitute about 13% of the population.

■ Individuals aged 65 and older account for the majority of cases of breast cancer and prostate cancer.

■ Advanced age is a risk factor for the development of cancer.

■ Older adults are more likely to be diagnosed with cancer at an advanced stage when the cancer is less amenable to treatment and increased morbidity and mortality are more likely.

■ Cancer diagnosis and mortality are strongly associated with race and socioeconomic status.

■ For both older men and women, lung cancer is the leading cause of mortality.

■ Lung cancer mortality rates are followed by prostate cancer and colorectal cancer for older men and breast cancer and colorectal cancer for older women.

■ Ageism and myths of aging prevented older adults from being involved in clinical trials for new cancer treatments; health care providers often perceived this population to be at high risk for adverse effects from the negative effects of cancer therapy.

■ More recently, older adults have begun to receive aggressive treatments for cancer and are tolerating these treatments well. Although special consideration for the normal and pathological changes of aging must be made, older adults should be offered the same treatments available to younger populations.

■ Nurses play an instrumental role in the primary and secondary prevention of cancer (see Chapter 5, "Health Promotion").

■ Providing support and information during the diagnosis is essential in treatment decision making and promoting effective cancer outcomes and quality of life.

Prostate Cancer

■ Of all men diagnosed with cancer each year, more than 30% will be diagnosed with prostate cancer.

■ This rate is higher for African Americans (American Cancer Society, 2015).

■ Prostate cancer is nearly 100% survivable if detected early (US Too! International, 2005–2015).

■ The availability of prostate-specific antigen testing for prostate cancer has greatly increased the detection and treatment of early-stage prostate tumors in older men.

■ Treatment for prostate cancer includes the options of:
  • Internal radiation (brachytherapy)
  • External beam radiation therapy
  • Radical prostatectomy

- Active surveillance or watchful waiting
- Hormonal therapy for late-stage disease

■ Nurses will be involved in administering treatments aimed at reducing the symptomatology surrounding this disease as well as aiding treatment.

Breast Cancer

■ 231,840 cases of breast cancer will be diagnosed in the United States in 2015, resulting in a projected 40,290 deaths.

■ Like prostate cancer in men, the risk of developing breast cancer increases with age among women.

■ Breast self-examination and mammography are helpful in screening for breast cancer.

■ The progression in lumpectomy and mastectomy procedures as well as new developments in radiation and chemotherapy treatments have sharply increased the survival rate for breast cancer for older women.

■ The nursing role in screening and administering treatments for breast cancer is essential in promoting good outcomes for these older women clients.

MUSCULOSKELETAL PROBLEMS

Osteoarthritis and Degenerative Joint Disease

■ Osteoarthritis (OA) is one of the most common chronic disorders among older adults.

■ OA is the number one cause of pain among older adults.

■ OA affects approximately 46.4 million Americans, 8.8% of whom report an arthritis-related disability (CDC, 2007b).

■ OA can be a primary disorder or a secondary disorder resulting from a previous anatomic abnormality, injury, or procedure or from occupational factors.

■ Nursing assessment for OA includes:
- The evaluation of pain because this is the presenting symptom for most patients
- Radiographic examination of the joints, which helps to aid in the diagnosis and staging of OA

▨ The nursing role for the treatment for OA is aimed at

- Relieving pain and preserving or restoring function

▨ Pharmacological treatments frequently include:

- NSAIDs

- Acetaminophen

- Narcotic pain relievers, when necessary

▨ Various complementary and alternative therapies aimed at reducing pain and improving function are used frequently by older adults with OA.

- Vitamins C, D, and E have shown some evidence of reducing symptoms.

- Ginger and glucosamine also have been used extensively by older adults to reduce arthritis-related pain.

- Nurses must exercise caution in the administration of nutraceuticals and provide instruction regarding the possible danger of taking these herbals with other medications because little is known about their interaction with prescription medications used to treat other diseases.

- Acupuncture is becoming a more popular nonpharmacological OA management strategy.

▨ Joint replacement among older adults with OA is gaining in popularity.

▨ Hip replacement surgery is common and greatly decreases pain and improves mobility among older adults.

- Prosthesis may become dislodged if early adduction of hip is sustained.

▨ These surgical procedures are used primarily to replace hip and knee joints that are dysfunctional because of the long-term effects of OA.

▨ Older individuals in their 80s and 90s typically have these procedures.

▨ Although the rehabilitation may be long and intense, joint replacement brings new mobility and has the potential to greatly improve quality of life.

Osteoporosis

Osteoporosis is one of the most common chronic diseases of older adulthood.

▨ Physiologically, osteoporosis results from a demineralization of the bone and is evidenced by a decrease in the mass and density of the skeleton.

▨ The most common areas of bone loss are the vertebrae, distal radius, and proximal femur.

▨ In older adults with osteoporosis, the overall decline in bone mass weakens the bone, making it vulnerable to even slight trauma.

■ Normal changes of aging in the sensory system and in neuromuscular coordination combine with medications and environmental factors to place older adults with osteoporosis at high risk for fall-related fractures.

■ Fractures of the humerus and femoral neck are common, as are hip fractures in women older than age 65.

  • Hip fractures result in greater morbidity and mortality among older adults than any other type of fracture.

■ Fractures in older adults often place these individuals in a spiral of iatrogenesis, with an increased risk of impaired mobility, pressure ulcers, pneumonia, and incontinence.

■ Older individuals who are at highest risk for osteoporosis include:

  • Small, thin women who have fair skin and light hair and eyes

  • Older adults with a family history of osteoporosis

  • Postmenopausal women

  • Women older than age 65

  • Men older than age 80

■ Older individuals are at greater risk if they

  • Have diets low in calcium

  • Smoke

  • Consume excess alcohol

  • Drink caffeine

  • Lead sedentary lifestyles

■ Older adults with osteoporosis may develop kyphosis late in the disease.

  • Kyphosis is a convex curvature of the spine that causes loss of height and chronic back pain as well as abdominal protuberance, gastrointestinal discomfort, and pulmonary insufficiency.

■ Bone density screenings can detect bone loss for those at risk for developing osteoporosis. However, because there are often no symptoms of this disease, osteoporosis is seldom diagnosed until a traumatic fracture is sustained.

■ Nursing interventions for the prevention of OA include:

  • Encouraging diets high in calcium (1,500 mg per day)

  • Advising a program of regular weight-bearing exercise

  • Medications that have been shown to prevent further bone loss in those diagnosed with osteoporosis; alendronate sodium (Fosamax) taken once a week or risedronate (Actonel) or raloxifene (Evista) have been shown to prevent further bone loss and develop new bone mass

  • Fall-prevention strategies (see Chapter 5)

METABOLIC AND ENDOCRINE PROBLEMS

Diabetes Mellitus

■ Diabetes mellitus (DM) is a chronic medical disease manifested by an increase in blood glucose levels.

■ The CDC (2015) reported that as of 2010, 10.9 million Americans age 65 or older have DM. It is the seventh leading cause of death in the United States.

■ DM is often a silent killer; it is estimated that 5.9 million Americans are unaware that they have the disease. Due to better screening and educational efforts at the state and national levels, diagnosis rates for diabetes have increased, and they are expected to continue to rise (Mokdad et al., 2001).

■ DM is a chronic metabolic disease characterized by a deficiency in the production and utilization of the pancreatic hormone insulin. In older adults, elevated blood glucose levels symptomatic of DM result from altered insulin availability.

■ There are two different types of DM: type 1 and type 2.

• Type 1 is also known as juvenile-onset DM or insulin-dependent DM.

• Type 2 DM generally appears during adulthood and is known as adult-onset DM or, more commonly, noninsulin-dependent diabetes mellitus (NIDDM).

■ DM is considered a risk factor for heart disease.

• More than 80% of persons with DM die of heart or blood vessel disease.

• Smoking drastically increases the risk of cardiovascular disease in diabetics by constricting already compromised blood vessels.

■ Nursing interventions for diabetes must begin with a thorough assessment of blood glucose values and HgA1C levels, which provide short- and long-term insulin function indicators.

■ The type of therapy should be tailored to the individual client's needs and issues.

■ Self-management of NIDDM in the elderly includes:

• Diet

• Medication

– Oral hypoglycemics

– Insulin therapy

• Blood glucose monitoring

• Foot examinations

• Exercise

IMMUNOLOGIC PROBLEMS

HIV/AIDS

■ 10% to 20% of HIV infections occur in people aged 50 and older.

■ This number is most likely low because of misdiagnosis and will continue to rise as the population of older adults grows.

■ Older adults progress from HIV to AIDS more quickly than younger adults because of normal and pathological aging changes.

■ Due to the normal and pathological changes of aging, symptoms of HIV and AIDS may go undetected.

■ The awareness of the possibility of STDs among older adults heightens the awareness of these potential disorders.

■ When sexual history questions lead the nurse to believe that the older adult is sexually active, especially with more than one partner, diagnostic testing should be conducted.

■ Symptoms of HIV among older adults mimic other disease symptoms and may include:

• Diarrhea

• Enlarged lymph nodes

• Fever

• Flulike symptoms

• Headache

• Rash

• Fatigue

• Anorexia

• Weight loss

■ Because HIV is often transmitted simultaneously with other STDs, the ELISA test may be used to diagnose the presence of HIV.

• If this test is positive, the Western blot test may be conducted to confirm HIV infection.

• Viral cultures may be used to confirm HIV infection.

• CD4 and viral load testing to measure the number of T helper cells helps to stage the disease.

■ Nursing interventions for older adults with HIV include:

• Maintenance of health and function

• Medication administration and teaching

• Antiretroviral agents and highly active antiretroviral agents (the use of three or more antiretroviral agents together)

- Nucleoside/nucleotide reverse transcriptase inhibitors
- Nonnucleoside reverse transcriptase inhibitors
- Protease inhibitors
- Fusion inhibitors
- Teaching safe-sex practices

NEUROLOGIC PROBLEMS

Parkinson's Disease

Parkinson's disease (PD) is one of the most common neurodegenerative disorders affecting the elderly population. It occurs in 1 of every 100 persons older than the age of 60.

■ It is estimated that 3% of persons older than the age of 65 have PD, suggesting that the occurrence of the disease increases with age.

■ PD affects men more than women and Whites more than Blacks or Asian Americans.

■ Age is the primary risk factor for PD and so the disease is of concern among older adults.

■ PD is a neurodegenerative disorder of slow and insidious onset, where 70% to 80% of the dopamine-producing neurons in the brain are destroyed by the time symptoms are present.

■ The causes of PD have not been determined.

- The roles of environmental toxins, poisons, viruses, and medications have been implicated in the development of PD, and these causes continue to be investigated.

- Some medications—including chlorpromazine and haloperidol as well as reserpine, methyldopa, and metoclopramide—have been linked to the development of PD symptoms.

■ There are no objective clinical markers for PD.

■ The diagnosis of PD is typically determined by the presence of these three motor signs:

- Tremor
- Rigidity
- Bradykinesia

■ In addition to these common signs and symptoms, clients with the disease may exhibit cues such as:

- Postural instability
- Autonomic dysfunction
- Drug-induced symptoms

■ Symptom management is the primary focus of nursing care. Psychological, social, and spiritual support are needed as the disease progresses.

- Treatment of PD generally combines levodopa with carbidopa (Sinemet).

- Because levodopa competes with protein absorption from the small intestine, effective timing of medication is essential.

- As symptoms progress, a client's ability to perform activities of daily living decreases and the need for pharmacotherapy increases.

- To avoid potential side effects, patients may choose nonpharmacological treatment options, delay medical treatment, and postpone potential discomfort from the unwanted side effects.

- Physical and occupational therapy may help those with a shuffling gait. Focusing on the client's balance abilities and providing assistive devices where applicable is recommended.

- Nutritional therapy is also essential when caring for patients with PD.

- Immobility is a major contributor to constipation; therefore, it is important to assess the dietary needs of PD clients to prevent severe constipation.

- Exercise is also extremely therapeutic for clients with PD. It decreases the risk of falls related to the disease and improves:
  - Mobility
  - Flexibility
  - Posture balance
  - Overall function

Cerebral Vascular Accident

■ CVAs, commonly known as strokes, are among the leading cause of chronic disability in the United States.

■ The risk of CVA increases sharply with age; approximately 75% of new strokes and 88% of stroke deaths occur among those aged 65 and older.

■ The symptoms of CVA include:

- Sudden-onset weakness or numbness in the face, leg, or arm on one side of the body

- Changes in vision; the loss of vision in one eye

- Difficulty speaking or understanding language

- Sudden-onset severe headache and dizziness

- Unexplained falls

■ Risk factors for the development of CVA are similar to those of other cardio-vascular diseases.

- Smoking
- Alcohol abuse
- Obesity
- Diabetes
- Hypertension
- Advanced age
- African American descent

■ CVAs are caused by three distinct pathological processes that stem from risk factors for the disease.

■ Effective auscultation of the carotid arteries for bruits (the sound of turbulent blood flow) during routine health assessments greatly enhances the early detection of occlusions in the vasculature and facilitates stroke prevention.

■ A hemorrhage results when a blood vessel in the brain ruptures and part of the brain tissue dies.

■ Emboli, or clots that form in one area of the body, may travel to the brain and cause brain death.

■ The carotid arteries that carry oxygenated blood to the brain may become clogged and prevent blood flow, resulting in tissue death (ischemia).

■ Older adults with and without risk factors for a CVA sometimes experience "little strokes" or warning strokes called TIAs.

- TIAs are manifested by lack of consciousness for a period of time lasting from 20 minutes to 24 hours.
- Reports of TIAs should be accompanied by a full assessment and the identification of risk factors and symptomatology for CVA.
- A plan of care to prevent strokes from occurring in patients with TIAs must be implemented immediately.

■ Prevention of CVAs generally involves the facilitation of adequate blood flow to the brain.

■ Carotid endarterectomy procedures are often implemented (cleaning plaque from the carotid artery) to enhance blood flow to the brain and reduce the chance of an embolus breaking off from the plaque and moving to the cerebral vasculature.

■ CVAs may be best prevented by implementing nursing interventions to reduce risk factors such as obesity and hypertension with

- Diet and nutritional management
- Exercise and weight reduction
- Blood pressure management
- Administration of daily aspirin

- When symptoms of a stroke are present, diagnostic testing is conducted, including:
  - Computed tomography scan
  - Carotid or cerebral angiography
  - Plasminogen activator, a clot-dissolving drug, may be administered immediately (within a few hours of symptom onset)
  - The plasminogen activator can dissolve clots that may have caused the stroke and quickly restore blood flow to the brain, but it is not effective in
    - Hemorrhagic stroke
    - Ischemic stroke
  - Nursing care for patients with CVA focuses on stabilization of the client and rehabilitation to the highest possible functional level

PRESSURE ULCERS

Pressure ulcers result from prolonged pressure to an area of the body. One million new pressure ulcers are estimated to develop each year.

- Both intrinsic and extrinsic risk factors result in the development of pressure ulcers, including:
  - Immobility (primary risk factor for development of pressure ulcers
  - Infection
  - Incontinence
  - Dementia
  - Malnutrition
  - Diabetes
  - Circulatory disorders
  - Vascular impairment
  - Edema
  - Impaired sensation
  - Transferring
  - High pressure surfaces
  - Sheering
  - Improper hygiene from poor nursing care
  - Circulation
- Pressure ulcers are classified according to the severity of the wound, usually in four stages or types (see Table 8.1)

TABLE 8.1   Pressure Ulcer Staging System

PRESSURE ULCER DEFINITION

A pressure ulcer is a localized injury to the skin and/or underlying tissue that usually occurs over a bony prominence, as a result of pressure or pressure in combination with shear and/or friction. A number of contributing or confounding factors are associated with pressure ulcers; the significance of these factors is yet to be elucidated.

PRESSURE ULCER STAGES

Suspected Deep-Tissue Injury

Purple or maroon localized areas of discolored intact skin or a blood-filled blister due to damage of underlying soft tissue from pressure and/or shear. The area may begin as tissue that is painful, firm, mushy, boggy, warmer, or cooler as compared to adjacent tissue.

Further description: Deep-tissue injury may be difficult to detect in individuals with dark skin. Evolution may include a thin blister over a dark wound bed. The wound may further evolve and become covered by thin eschar. Evolution may be rapid, exposing additional layers of tissue even with optimal treatment.

Stage I

Intact skin with nonblanchable redness of a localized area usually over a bony prominence. Darkly pigmented skin may not have visible blanching, but its color may differ from the surrounding area.

Further description: The area may be painful, firm, soft, warmer, or cooler as compared to adjacent tissue. Stage I may be difficult to detect in individuals with dark skin. May indicate at-risk persons (a heralding sign of risk).

Stage II

Partial-thickness loss of dermis presenting as a shallow open ulcer with a red–pink wound bed, without slough. May also present as an intact or open/ruptured serum-filled blister.

Further description: Presents as a shiny or dry shallow ulcer without slough or bruising.* This stage should not be used to describe skin tears, tape burns, perineal dermatitis, maceration, or excoriation.

Stage III

Full-thickness tissue loss. Subcutaneous fat may be visible, but bone, tendon, or muscle is not exposed. Slough may be present but does not obscure the depth of tissue loss. May include undermining and tunneling.

Further description: The depth of a stage III pressure ulcer varies by anatomical location. The bridge of the nose, ear, occiput, and malleolus do not have subcutaneous tissue. And stage III ulcers can be shallow. In contrast, areas of significant adiposity can develop extremely deep stage III pressure ulcers. Bone/tendon is not visible or directly palpable.

Stage IV

Full-thickness tissue loss with exposed bone, tendon, or muscle. Slough or eschar may be present on some parts of the wound bed. Often includes undermining and tunneling.

Further description: The depth of a stage IV pressure ulcer varies by anatomical location. The bridge of the nose, ear, occiput, and malleolus do not have subcutaneous tissue and these ulcers can be shallow. Stage IV ulcers can extend into muscle and/or supporting structures (e.g., fascia, tendon, or joint capsule) making osteomyelitis possible. Exposed bone/tendon is visible or directly palpable.

Unstageable

Full-thickness loss in which the base of the ulcer is covered by slough (yellow, tan, gray, green, or brown) and/or eschar (tan, brown, or black) in the wound bed.

Further description: Until enough slough and/or eschar is removed to expose the base of the wound, the true depth; therefore, the ulcer's stage cannot be determined. Stable (dry, adherent, intact without erythema or fluctuance) eschar on the heels serves as the body's natural (biological) cover and should not be removed.

Note: *Bruising indicates suspected deep-tissue injury.

From National Pressure Ulcer Advisory Panel (2007). European Pressure Ulcer Advisory Panel and Pan Pacific Pressure Injury Alliance. Copyright 2014, used with permission.

■ The most effective nursing intervention for pressure ulcers is prevention

■ Assessment of risk factors (see Table 8.2) enables nurses to identify and implement preventative measures to avoid the development of these wounds

■ Preventative measures include:

- The use of pressure-relieving devices such as

  - Mattresses

  - Pads

  - Footwear

- Proper body alignment—"Rule of 30," or head of bed elevated 30 degrees

- Regular and consistent skin assessment by knowledgeable nursing professionals with a reliable instrument will help to detect pressure ulcers at an early, treatable stage

- Turning and repositioning schedules

- Eliminating risk factors for malnutrition and create appropriate meal planning

- Dietary supplements may be necessary for providing needed nutrition among chronically ill older adults

■ Pressure ulcer treatments include:

- Daily care with recommended products is implemented according to wound stage.

  - Stage I ulcers (nonblanchable erythema) are protected from further damage with good hygiene and pressure relief; transparent dressings may be used.

  - Stage II ulcers are characterized by partial-thickness skin loss involving epidermis, dermis, or both and generally are treated with occlusive dressings and reevaluated at regular intervals.

  - Stage III ulcers are characterized by full-thickness skin loss and deep craters with or without undermining; utilize normal saline or other product dressings.

SENSORY PROBLEMS

Common Eye Diseases

Cataracts

■ Result from accumulation of particles in the lens of the eye

■ Have great impact on vision

■ Previously had been untreatable

■ Laser procedures to clear the lens and return vision to normal can be completed in approximately 1 hour and have few side effects

TABLE 8.2 Braden Scale for Predicting Pressure Sore Risk

PATIENT'S NAME _____ EVALUATOR'S NAME _____ DATE OF ASSESSMENT _____

	1	2	3	4
Sensory Perception Ability to respond meaningfully to pressure-related discomfort	**1. Completely Limited** Unresponsive (does not moan, flinch, or grasp) due to painful stimuli, due to diminished level of consciousness or sedation. OR Limited ability to feel pain over most of body.	**2. Very Limited** Responds only to painful stimuli. Cannot communicate discomfort except by moaning or restlessness. OR Has a sensory impairment that limits the ability to feel pain or discomfort over half of body.	**3. Slightly Limited** Responds to verbal commands but cannot always communicate discomfort or the need to be turned. OR Has some sensory impairment that limits ability to feel pain or discomfort in one or two extremities.	**4. No Impairment** Responds to verbal commands. Has no sensory deficit that would limit ability to feel or voice pain or discomfort.
Moisture Degree to which skin is exposed to moisture	**1. Constantly Moist** Skin is kept moist almost constantly by perspiration, urine, etc. Dampness is detected every time patient is moved or turned.	**2. Very Moist** Skin is often, but not always, moist. Linen must be changed at least once a shift.	**3. Occasionally Moist** Skin is occasionally moist, requiring an extra linen change approximately once a day.	**4. Rarely Moist** Skin is usually dry, linen only requires changing at routine intervals.
Activity Degree of physical activity	**1. Bedfast** Confined to bed.	**2. Chairfast** Ability to walk severely limited or nonexistent. Cannot bear own weight and/or must be assisted into chair or wheelchair.	**3. Walks Occasionally** Walks occasionally during day, but for very short distances, with or without assistance. Spends majority of each shift in bed or chair.	**4. Walks Frequently** Walks outside room at least twice a day and inside room at least once every 2 hours during waking hours.
Mobility Ability to change and control body position	**1. Completely Immobile** Does not make even slight changes in body or extremity position without assistance.	**2. Very Limited** Makes occasional slight changes in body or extremity position but unable to make frequent or significant changes independently.	**3. Slightly Limited** Makes frequent though slight changes in body or extremity position independently.	**4. No Limitation** Makes major and frequent changes in position without assistance.

	1. Very Poor	2. Probably Inadequate	3. Adequate	4. Excellent
Nutrition Usual food intake pattern	Never eats a complete meal. Rarely eats more than one third of any food offered. Eats two servings or less of protein (meat or dairy products) per day. Takes fluids poorly. Does not take a liquid dietary supplement. OR Is NPO and/or maintained on clear liquids or IVs for more than 5 days.	Rarely eats a complete meal and generally eats only about half of any food offered. Protein intake includes only three servings of meat or dairy products per day. Occasionally will take a dietary supplement. OR Receives less than optimum amount of liquid diet or tube feeding.	Eats over half of most meals. Eats a total of four servings of protein (meat, dairy products) per day. Occasionally will refuse a meal, but will usually take a supplement when offered. OR Is on a tube-feeding or TPN regimen, which probably meets most nutritional needs.	Eats most of every meal. Never refuses a meal. Usually eats a total of four or more servings of meat and dairy products. Occasionally eats between meals. Does not require supplementation.
	1. Problem	2. Potential Problem	3. No Apparent Problem	
Friction and Shear	Requires moderate to maximum assistance in moving. Complete lifting without sliding against sheets is impossible. Frequently slides down in bed or chair, requiring frequent repositioning with maximum assistance. Spasticity, contractures, or agitation leads to almost constant friction.	Moves feebly or requires minimum assistance. During a move, skin probably slides to some extent against sheets, chair, restraints, or other devices. Maintains relatively good position in chair or bed most of the time but occasionally slides down.	Moves in bed and in chair independently and has sufficient muscle strength to lift up completely during move. Maintains good position in bed or chair.	

Score: 15–18 at risk; 13–14 moderate risk; 10–12 high risk; > 9 very high risk. Total Score:

NPO, nothing by mouth; IV, intravenously; TPN, total parenteral nutrition.

From Braden and Bergstrom (1988). Copyright ©. All rights reserved.

Glaucoma

■ Results from a pathological accumulation of pressure in the internal chamber of the eye

■ Requires the consistent use of pressure-relieving eye drops

■ Lower levels of lighting may be needed to promote patient comfort

■ Regular ophthalmological appointments for pressure readings are essential

■ Surgical interventions are available when necessary

Common Ear Disease: Presbycusis

■ High-pitched hearing loss that occurs commonly with aging.

■ Makes it difficult to hear high-pitched voices, such as those of women and children.

■ Treatment is usually associated with amplifying sound with hearing aids.

  • Older adults sometimes do not like hearing aids because they are embarrassed about needing them and because they amplify all noises in the environment, further aggravating the hearing deficit.

  • Assess for cerumen impaction as a further complicating factor in the hearing impaired.

  • Face older adults when speaking to facilitate lip reading.

  • Do not shout.

  • Assess for the appropriateness of using alternate forms of communication, such as writing instructions.

REFERENCES

Alliance for Aging Research. (2002). *Medical never-never land.* Retrieved from http://www.agingresearch.org/content/article/detail1698

American Cancer Society. (2015). *Overview: Prostate cancer, how many men get prostate cancer?* Retrieved from http://www.cancer.org/docroot/CRI/content/CRI_2_2_1X_How_many_men_get_prostate_cancer_36.asp?sitearea=

American Heart Association. (2015). *Heart disease and stroke statistics.* 2005 update. Retrieved from http://www.americanheart.org/downloadedheart/

American Heart Association. (2013). *Facts about women and cardiovascular diseases.* Retrieved from http://www.americanheart.org/presenter.jhtml?identifier=2876

Annon, J. (1976). The PLISSIT model: A proposed conceptual scheme for the behavioral treatment for sexual problems. *Journal of Sex Education Therapy*, 2(2), 1–15.

Beers, M. H., & Berkow, R. (Eds.). (2000). *Merck manual of geriatrics* (3rd ed.). Whitehouse Station, NJ: Merck Research Laboratories.

Braden, B., & Bergstrom, N. (1988). *Braden scale.* Retrieved from http://www.bradenscale.com

Centers for Disease Control and Prevention. (2005). *Highlights in minority health, November 2003: National diabetes awareness month.* Retrieved from http://www.cdc .gov/omhd/High lights/2002&3/HNov03.htm

Centers for Disease Control and Prevention. (2007a). *Key facts about the flu.* Retrieved July 18, 2007, from http://www.cdc.gov/flu/keyfacts.htm

Centers for Disease Control and Prevention. (2007b). *Arthritis data and statistics.* Retrieved from http://www.cdc.gov/arthritis/data_statistics/index.htm

Centers for Disease Control and Prevention. (2013). *State indicator report on fruits and vegetables, 2013.* Atlanta, GA: The Centers for Disease Control and Prevention, U.S. Department of Health and Human Services. Retrieved from http://www .cdc.gov/nutrition/downloads/State-Indicator-Report-Fruits-Vegerables-2013.pdf

Institute for Clinical Systems Improvement. (2006). *Health care guideline: Community acquired pneumonia in adults.* Retrieved from http://www.icsi.org

Miller, S. K. (2007). Getting a grip on GERD. *American Nurse Today, 2*(6), 12–14.

Mokdad, A. H., Bowman, B. A., Ford, E. S., Vinicor, F., Marks, J. S., & Koplan, J. P. (2001). The continuing epidemics of obesity and diabetes in the United States. *Journal of the American Medical Association, 286,* 1195–1200.

National Pressure Ulcer Advisory Panel. (2007). *Updated pressure ulcer staging 2007.* Retrieved from http://www.npuap.org/pr2.htm

Ward, B. W., Schiller, J. S., Goodman, R. A. (2014). Multiple chronic conditions among US adults: A 2012 update. *Preventing Chronic Disease, 11,* E62. dx.doi.org/10.5888/ pcd11.130389

Web Site Icon. Us Too! International. (2005–2015). *Informed brochure.* Retrieved from http://www. ustoo.org

9

Cognitive and Psychological Disorders

DEPRESSION AND SUICIDE

- The frequent experience of loss among the elderly was once used to explain the large incidence of depression among older adults.
- Men who are 65 and older are among the highest risk groups for suicide (Centers for Disease Control and Prevention, 2014).
- Transitions may play a role in the development of depression but are not usually the only cause. Such transitions include:
  - Retirement
  - Relocation
  - Loss of spouse, friends, and family
  - Financial constraints
  - Illness
- Recent research on depression indicates that there is more to the development of depression than the experience of loss.
- The role of neurotransmitters in the development of depression among older adults also contributes to the development of depression in this population.
- Medication use can also be a contributing factor in the development of depression. Drug classes frequently implicated in the development of depressive symptoms include: antihypertensives, cardiac medications, hormones, analgesics, sedatives, and anxiolytics.
- The pathophysiology of certain conditions, such as hypothyroidism and malnutrition, can result in depression.
- Chronic, unrelieved pain significantly increases the risk of depression and suicide.
- Because of the many physiological changes that accompany aging, older adults are more susceptible to the effects of altered neurotransmission than any other age group.

▪ Older adults have the highest rate of depression, and the rate is even higher among older adults with coexisting medical conditions.

▪ 12% of older persons hospitalized for problems such as hip fracture or heart disease are diagnosed with depression. Treating depression in these patients improves the long-term outcomes of these patients and results in reduced mortality.

▪ Rates of depression for older people in nursing homes range from 15% to 25%

▪ Genetic factors may be significant because depression is often seen in members of the same family

▪ Women have a higher incidence of depression than men, although men have a higher suicide rate

▪ There is a strong correlation between alcohol or drug abuse and depression, not only in the client but also in his or her family

▪ Unmarried individuals with low support networks are at high risk for depression

▪ Assessment for depression in older adults should include:

  • A complete history, including family history and suicide attempts

  • Completion of a depression scale such as the Geriatric Depression Scale (see Table 9.1)

TABLE 9.1   Geriatric Depression Scale: Short Form

A. Five (or more) of the following symptoms have been present during the same 2-week period and represent a change from previous functioning; at least one of the symptoms is either (1) depressed mood or (2) loss of interest or pleasure. (*Note:* Do not include symptoms that are clearly caused by a general medical condition or mood-incongruent delusions or hallucinations.)

1. Depressed mood most of the day, nearly every day, as indicated by either subjective report (e.g., feels sad or empty) or observation made by others (e.g., appears tearful). Note: In children and adolescents, can be irritable mood.
2. Markedly diminished interest or pleasure in all, or almost all, activities most of the day, nearly every day (as indicated by either subjective account or observation made by others).
3. Significant weight loss when not dieting or weight gain (e.g., a change of more than 5% of body weight in a month) or decrease or increase in appetite nearly every day. (Note: In children, consider failure to make expected weight gains.)
4. Insomnia or hypersomnia nearly every day.
5. Psychomotor agitation or retardation nearly every day (observable by others, not merely subjective feelings of restlessness or being slowed down).
6. Fatigue or loss of energy nearly every day.
7. Feelings of worthlessness or excessive or inappropriate guilt (which may be delusional) nearly every day (not merely self-reproach or guilt about being sick).
8. Diminished ability to think or concentrate or indecisiveness nearly every day (either by subjective account or as observed by others).
9. Recurrent thoughts of death (not just fear of dying), recurrent suicidal ideation without a specific plan, or a suicide attempt or a specific plan for committing suicide.

(continued)

TABLE 9.1 Geriatric Depression Scale: Short Form (*continued*)

B. The symptoms do not meet criteria for a mixed episode.
C. The symptoms cause clinically significant distress or impairment in social, occupational, or other important areas of functioning.
D. The symptoms are not due to the direct physiological effects of a substance (e.g., a drug of abuse or a medication) or a general medical condition (e.g., hypothyroidism).
E. The symptoms are not better accounted for by bereavement (i.e., after the loss of a loved one); the symptoms persist for longer than 2 months; or are characterized by marked functional impairment, morbid preoccupation with worthlessness, suicidal ideation, psychotic symptoms, or psychomotor retardation.

From Aging Clinical Research Center, Stanford University (2015).

- In addition to the possibility of suicide, complications of depression include:
  - Amplification of pain
  - Delayed recovery from surgery and illness
  - Cognitive impairment
  - Malnutrition
- Treatment options for depression include both psychotherapy and pharmacotherapy. The various treatment options may be combined or used individually.
- Psychotherapy led by mental health professionals includes:
  - Individual talk therapy
  - Family therapy
  - Group therapy
- Medication options include:
  - Selective serotonin reuptake inhibitors (SSRIs): fluoxetine (Prozac), paroxetine (Paxil), and sertraline (Zoloft)
    - SSRIs are a class of medications that work by inhibiting the reuptake of serotonin, thus increasing its concentration in the space between nerve cells.
    - These antidepressant medications have an overall lower side-effect profile than their predecessor antidepressants, but they are not perfect.
    - The most common side effects of SSRIs are
      - Nausea
      - Diarrhea
      - Insomnia
      - Dry mouth
      - Tremors
    - SSRIs are usually given in the morning right after breakfast

- Recent reports on SSRIs have shown that clients with Parkinson's disease (and possibly other tremor disorders) may experience exacerbations of their condition to the point of inducing Parkinsonian crisis.
- Tricyclic antidepressants (TCAs): amitriptyline (Elavil), imipramine (Tofranil), and nortriptyline (Pamelor)
  - TCAs are among the oldest forms of antidepressants.
  - They work by blocking the reuptake of various neurotransmitters, such as norepinephrine and serotonin.
  - This action allows the chemicals to remain in the synaptic junction (the space between the neurons) for a longer period of time.
  - The presence of these neurotransmitters aids the feeling of well-being.
  - TCAs are associated with the following side effects:
    ○ Dry mouth
    ○ Constipation
    ○ Tremors
    ○ Blurred vision
    ○ Postural hypotension
    ○ Sedation
    ○ Urinary retention
    ○ Because some of these side effects increase the client's risk for falls, they are usually administered just before bedtime
    ○ It is also essential that clients on these medications be placed on a fall-prevention program
- Monoamine oxidase inhibitors (MAOIs): phenelzine (Nardil) and tranylcypromine (Parnate)
  - MAOIs are seldom used in older adults because they have a high risk of very significant side effects in this population.
  - They work by blocking various subtypes of monoamine oxidase, which is the chemical responsible for breaking down norepinephrine, serotonin, and dopamine.
  - Like the TCAs, these chemicals remain in the neuroleptic synapse.
  - Common side effects of MAOIs:
    ○ Orthostatic hypotension
    ○ Tachycardia
    ○ Edema
    ○ Dizziness
    ○ Agitation

- It is imperative that clients taking MAOIs follow a strict diet low in tyramines (found in aged cheeses, for example) and avoid certain medications (such as those containing ergotamine).
- Failure to follow these restrictions could precipitate a hypertensive crisis that is potentially life threatening (Bernstein, 1995).
- Atypical antidepressants do not fall into a specific drug category.
  - Trazodone (Desyrel) inhibits serotonin reuptake
  - Bupropion (Wellbutrin) is a mild blocker of the reuptake of dopamine, norepinephrine, and serotonin.
  - Side effects for both include:
    ○ Dry mouth
    ○ Dizziness
    ○ Drowsiness
    ○ Nausea
    ○ Vomiting
    ○ Increased risk of seizures
  - Electroconvulsive therapy (ECT)
    ○ ECT is used in clients who have severe treatment-resistant depression.
    ○ ECT is not the usual first-line treatment for depression at any age.
    ○ Older adults may experience more memory loss for a period of time after the treatment.

RELATIONSHIP OF DEPRESSION AND SUICIDAL IDEATION

- The depressed client has an increased risk of suicidal ideation.
- Approximately 15% of severely depressed people commit suicide.
- Depressed people have 30 times the suicide risk compared to the general population.
- Suicide among older adults is particularly common.
- People age 65 and older account for 12% of the population, but they commit almost 20% of all suicides.
- Women make more suicide attempts, but men complete their attempts three times more often.
- Suicidal ideation is the phrase used to describe the thought process of thinking about suicide.
- Nurses should ask specifically whether the client is thinking of hurting or killing himself or herself.
- Research has shown that 80% of people who have committed suicide told someone about it first, often a primary care provider.

- If a person talks about suicide, he or she has active suicidal ideation, and action must be taken immediately.
- One should never leave a person with active suicidal ideation alone.
- If the person is not an inpatient, he or she should be taken to the nearest psychiatric center or emergency department.
- If an older adult refuses to go to the emergency department, the legal system has several options to help protect the suicidal person—call 911.
- If a suicide attempt appears imminent, the client is put on constant one-to-one monitoring.
- The client's primary health care professional should be notified immediately so that the need for drug therapy can be evaluated and initiated if indicated.
- All items that could be potentially used by the client to cause injury should be removed. These items include:
  - Razors
  - Jewelry with pins or sharp points
  - Belts
  - Shoelaces
  - Eating utensils
  - Mirrors
  - Nails used to hang pictures on the walls
  - Nail files
  - Medications
  - Aerosol sprays
  - Paint

DEMENTIA

- Decline in the cognitive function of older adults is a prevalent concern and a focus of study in the older population.
- Although normal changes of aging result in a decrease in brain weight and a shift in the proportion of gray matter to white matter, the development of dementia is not a normal change of aging.
- *Dementia* is a general term used to describe over 60 pathological cognitive disorders that occur as a result of
  - Disease
  - Heredity
  - Lifestyle
  - Environmental influences

■ Dementia has underlying organic causes, including:

- Vascular disease

- Central nervous system infections

- Cortical degeneration

- Brain trauma

- Metabolic or toxic disorders

- Neurological disorders such as, Alzheimer's disease (AD) or Parkinson's disease

■ There is a difference between normal forgetfulness, which can happen at any age, and dementia.

■ Dementia is a chronic loss of cognitive function that progresses over a long period of time.

Dementia, as defined by the Alzheimer's Association, is a "loss of mental function in two or more areas such as language, memory, visual and spatial abilities, or judgment severe enough to interfere with daily life" (p. 8).

■ Here is a commonly used scenario to discriminate between normal memory loss and dementia: If you lose your car keys, you simply experienced memory loss. If you find them and don't know what they are for, you have a more serious cognitive problem.

■ Essential features of dementia include short- and long-term memory loss associated with impairment in construct thinking, impaired judgment, and other disturbances of higher cortical function that may result in personality change, which may be manifested in

- Difficulty coping with new situations

- Excessive motor or verbal activity

  - Irritability

  - Restlessness

  - Hyperactivity

  - Wandering

■ Patients experiencing cognitive impairment should be approached slowly, with care, and compassion in order to avoid resistance to care. If patients are resisting nursing care, an attempt should be made to understand whether there are factors causing the resistance, such as untreated pain.

■ AD is the most common type of dementia, making up over 50% of dementia cases.

- The cause of AD is not known.

- Two risk factors for the development of AD are

  - Advanced age

  - Family history of the disease

■ Ten early warning signs of AD are
- Misplacing items
- Loss of initiative
- Changes in personality
- Poor judgment
- Changes in mood or behavior
- Disorientation to time and place
- Memory loss that affects job skills
- Difficulty performing familiar tasks
- Difficulty finding the right words
- Problems with abstract thinking

■ Assessment of cognitive function to diagnose dementia:
- A standardized cognitive assessment instrument, such as the Mini-Cog (see Figure 4.1 in Chapter 4), can be used.
- Definitive diagnosis of all but multi-infarct dementia formerly was limited to postmortem brain autopsy.
- If older adults score low on screening instruments for cognitive impairments, they should be evaluated
  - for a comprehensive geriatric assessment to aide in the diagnosis of AD
  - to rule out delirium, depression, and other possible causes of altered cognitive status
- Assessments and care may need to be stopped to facilitate patient comfort and safety.
- The focus is on maintaining function and independence as much as possible, while keeping the older adult safe.
- Nurses who work with older adults are developing interventions to increase the quality of life for those who suffer from dementia.
- These interventions include:
  - Maintaining familiar environments to keep patients comfortable and safe
  - Necessary environmental manipulations such as camouflaging doors and installing door alarms
  - Applying "wander guards"
  - Providing safe wandering areas

■ The Alzheimer's Association (2006) recommends the techniques shown in Table 9.2 for caring for older adults with dementia.

■ Several medications known as cholinesterase inhibitors have been developed to increase the levels of acetylcholine in the brain and prevent further loss of cognitive function. These medications include:

- Donepezil (Aricept)
- Galantamine (Reminyl)
- Rivastigmine (Exelon)
- Tacrine (Cognex)

■ Namenda, or memantine, differs from the cholinesterase inhibitors

TABLE 9.2 Tips for Caring for Older Adults With Dementia

ASSESS	INTERVENE	EVALUATE
Identify the troublesome behaviors	**Explore potential solutions**	**Did your intervention help?**
■ What was the behavior?	■ Are there unmet needs of the person with dementia—is he or she sick, in pain, or sexually unfulfilled?	■ Do you need to explore other potential causes and solutions to the behavior?
■ What happened just before or after the behavior? Did something trigger it?	■ Can you adapt the environment instead of the person?	
■ What was your reaction?	■ Can you change your reaction or approach to the behavior?	

Adapted from Alzheimer's Association (2006).

DELIRIUM

■ *Delirium* is defined as a transient state of global cognitive impairment (Foreman, 1993).

- Reduced ability to maintain attention to external stimuli and to shift appropriate attention to new external stimuli
- Disorganized thinking
- At least two of the following:
  - Reduced level of consciousness
  - Perceptual disturbances
  - Disturbance of the sleep–wake cycle
  - Increased or decreased psychomotor behavior
  - Disorientation to person, place, or time
  - Memory impairment

■ These symptoms of delirium, commonly thought of as acute confusion, usually develop over a short period of time.

■ Estimates of the incidence and prevalence of delirium in acute care settings show that approximately 16% of older adults experience this short-term cognitive disorder.

- Delirium is not a disease as much as a syndrome that may result from a variety of causes.
- The specific symptoms of delirium that separate it from dementia are
  - Acute onset
  - Fluctuating course
- Delirium may develop in both cognitively intact and cognitively impaired older adults.
- The cause of delirium is not fully known.
- Suggested risk factors for the onset of delirium are:
  - Previous brain pathology
  - Decreased ability to manage change
  - Impaired sensory function
  - Presence of acute and chronic diseases
  - Changes in medications
  - Translocation
  - Cognitive impairment
  - Sensory impairment or deprivation
  - Co-morbidity
  - Depression
  - Alcohol use
  - Physical restraints
  - Malnutrition
  - Administration of more than three medications
  - Urinary catheterization
  - Iatrogenic events
- Delirium has vast implications for older adults, their families, and the U.S. economy, including:
  - Increased hospital stays
  - Failure to assess underlying and causative disease processes
- Prevention of delirium by risk factor minimization is essential.
- If delirium is assessed, treatment includes:
  - Identifying and removing the cause
  - Keeping the older adult safe
  - Implementing fall and wandering interventions
  - Avoiding the use of restraints (physical and chemical) because this may exacerbate the delirium

- Maintaining nutrition and hydration status
- Providing a calm, soft-spoken approach to care
- Frequently reassuring families of the temporary nature of this syndrome

REFERENCES

Aging Clinical Research Center, Stanford University. (2015). Retrieved from http://www.stanford.edu/~yesavage/GDS.html

Alzheimer's Association. (2015). *2015, Alzheimer's disease facts and figures*. Retrieved from http://www.alz.org/facts/overview/asp

Alzheimer's Association. (2006). *Behaviors*. Retrieved from http://www.alz.org/national/documents/brochure_behaviors.pdf

Bernstein, J. A. (1995). Nonimmunologic adverse drug reactions: How to recognize and categorize some common reactions. *Postgraduate Medicine, 98*, 120–126.

Centers for Disease Control and Prevention. (2014). *National suicide statistics at a gance*. Retrieved from http://www.cdc.gov/violenceprevention/suicide/statistics/trends03.html

Foreman, M. D. (1993). Acute confusion in the elderly. *Annual Review of Nursing Research, 11*, 3–30.

Puentes, W. J. (2002). Simple reminiscence: A stress-adaptation model of the phenomenon. *Issues in Mental Health Nursing, 23*(5), 497–511.

10

Medication

POLYPHARMACY

- More than half of older adults take five or more prescription and over-the-counter medications daily (Qato et al., 2008).

- The availability of multiple and effective medications to treat the numerous diseases prevalent among older adults undoubtedly plays an instrumental role in the increasing life span of this population.

- As older adults age, the number of prescription medications used increases.

- 68% of older adults taking prescription medications also take one or more over-the-counter medications, increasing the likelihood of drug–drug interactions. Research has found that one of the most common drug–drug interactions is the interaction between Coumadin (warfarin) and aspirin (Qato et al., 2008). When these two medications are taken together, the risk of bleeding and stroke increases substantially.

BEERS CRITERIA

The Beers criteria outline a list of medications that may be potentially inappropriate in older adults. These medications often have side-effect profiles, which are heightened with age, and therefore need to be used with caution in older adults. Although the list does not suggest an absolute contraindication against the use of these medications, they should not be used as first-line agents, and their use requires careful monitoring. The major categories of inappropriate medications include (a) those with significant side effects or limited benefits, (b) those that may exacerbate illness, and (c) those that should be administered with caution in older adults.

PHARMACOKINETICS AND PHARMACODYNAMICS

- Pharmacokinetics is the study of drug absorption, distribution, protein

■ Pharmacodynamics is the study of drug effects at the receptor level.
■ Normal changes of aging and pathological illness often influence pharmacokinetics and pharmacodynamics among older adults. These changes are summarized in Table 10.1.
■ The four pharmacokinetic mechanisms—absorption, distribution, metabolism, and elimination—are also influenced by acute and chronic illnesses common in older adulthood, which may further slow or impair the ability of organ systems to absorb, distribute, metabolize, and excrete medications.
■ These changes affect how medications are absorbed through the gastrointestinal track, skin, or musculature.
■ Although older adults experience many anatomical and physiological changes throughout life, there is currently little evidence to support the notion that normal aging significantly impacts drug absorption.
■ Nutritional deficiencies are prevalent among older adults.
■ Conditions that may impact drug absorption include:

• Achlorhydria, a disease that reduces the acidity of the stomach, which may make it difficult to dissolve medications for absorption

• Gastroesophageal reflux disease

• Surgery to the stomach or small intestine

TABLE 10.1 Pharmacokinetic Changes With Aging

PHARMACOKINETICS	CHANGES IN OLDER ADULTS
Drug absorption	■ Increase in gastric pH and a change in the amount of fluid in the stomach ■ Decrease in time required to empty stomach contents ■ Takes stomach longer to move nutrients across the membrane ■ Increase in time needed for medications to become effective ■ Increase in time may also increase amount of medication absorbed ■ Vitamins A and C may be more readily absorbed
Drug distribution	■ Reduced lean body mass ■ Increased percentage of body fat ■ Altered plasma protein binding ■ Decline in cardiac output by 1% every year ■ Decline in blood flow to the liver from 0.3% to 1.5% a year
Drug metabolism	■ Reduced blood flow to the liver ■ Decreased number of functional liver cells ■ Reduced number of enzymes used to break down medicines
Drug elimination	■ Reduced mass and reduced number and size of the nephrons ■ Reduced glomerular filtration rate ■ Decreased renal tubular secretion

■ Drugs are distributed via the circulatory system
- Total body intracellular and extracellular water decreases by as much as 15% among older adults.
- This reduces the distribution of water-soluble medications and increases the amount of fat-soluble medications.
- Lean body mass is reduced in older adults.
- The proportion of fat tissue increases with age from 18% to 36% in men and from 36% to 48% in women between the ages of 20 and 80.
- Fat-soluble medications such as barbiturates, phenothiazines, benzodiazepines, and phenytoin have the tendency to accumulate in the increased fat distribution of older adults, resulting in a prolonged half-life of these medications.
- Alterations in plasma protein binding that may occur as part of the normal aging process could alter the distribution of a medication significantly, as well as change the half-life of a medication and disrupt the steady flow of medication needed for disease management.
- Cardiac output, which declines by about 1% each year after the age of 30, has the potential to alter medication distribution.
- Pathological illness affecting the circulatory system (i.e., diabetes) may impact medication distribution.

■ Drugs are metabolized by the bodily organ systems
- Although medication metabolism depends on adequate liver function, that function is difficult to determine.
- In the absence of diagnosed liver disease, it can be challenging to predict how medications will be metabolized among the elderly.
- The following factors potentially affect liver function and reduce the metabolism of medications.
  - Multiple medications
  - Alcohol use
  - Caffeine use
  - Smoking
  - Poor nutrition
  - Multiple disease processes

■ Drugs are eliminated from the body through the kidneys
- Elimination of medications among older adults is one of the most well-studied and predictable age-related changes in medication pharmacokinetics.
- Creatinine clearance is not the most reliable measure of renal function and elimination of medications among older adults.
- A more sensitive measure of medication elimination of older adults incor-

ADVERSE DRUG REACTIONS AND SIDE EFFECTS

■ Changes of aging and pharmacodynamics as well as the presence of disease and the numerous prescription and over-the-counter drugs taken by older adults (polypharmacy) put this population at high risk for developing adverse reactions to drugs.

■ Older adults are estimated to be at two to three times higher risk for adverse reactions to medications than their younger counterparts.

■ Drug–drug interactions

- Drug–drug interactions are defined as the combination of two or more drugs such that the potency or efficacy of one drug is significantly modified by the presence of another.

■ Drug–disease interactions

- Older adults with certain diseases may have drug intolerance, such as:
  - Hypertension
  - Congestive heart failure
  - Diabetes
  - Renal failure
- These drug–disease interactions may necessitate discontinuation of a medication or finding an alternative that does not impact other disease processes.

■ Drug–nutrient interactions

- Drugs have been shown to impact the nutritional status of older adults in the following ways.
  - Medications tend to impact appetite.
  - Medications may affect the absorption, distribution, metabolism, and elimination of nutrients.
  - Nutrients may impact the absorption, distribution, metabolism, and elimination of drugs.
- Older adults are at higher risk for drug–nutrient interactions because of
  - Normal and pathological aging changes
  - Higher rates of alcoholism among the elderly
  - Use of restricted diets to treat disease
  - Use of nutritional supplements
- Administering medications via tube feedings creates a risk of drug–nutrient interactions.
- Certain nutrients are excreted more quickly if they interact with medications such as diuretics (e.g., thiazide).
- To reduce the risk of drug–nutrient interactions, medications should be administered with water.

COMPLIANCE ISSUES

■ About half of all patients take their medications as prescribed upon leaving the physician's office. The other half take the medications incorrectly or not at all.

■ Reasons for noncompliance with medication regimens include:
- Failure of health care professionals to give clear instructions on use of the medication
- Inability to afford medication
- Inability to understand complex medication dosing
- Conflicting beliefs about healing

■ Nursing interventions that may be helpful in enhancing medication adherence include:
- Assessment of understanding and beliefs regarding medications
- Teaching regarding the recommended treatment regimen
- The use of containers that are easily opened
- Bold labeling of medications

REFERENCE

Qato, D. M., Alexander, G. C., Conti, R. M., Johnson, M., Schumm, P., & Lindau, S. T. (2008). Use of prescription and over-the-counter medications and dietary supplements among older adults in the United States. *Journal of the American Medical Association*, 300(24), 2867–2878. doi:10.1001/jama.2008.892

11

Special Issues

PAIN

- Pain is a major problem for older adults and those who care for them.
- Pain has major implications for older adult health, functioning, and quality of life.
- Flaherty (2007) reports that 25% to 50% of community-dwelling older adults and 45% to 85% of nursing home residents have untreated pain.
- The number one cause of chronic pain among older adults is osteoarthritis.
- Chronic, untreated pain results in poor outcomes, such as:
  - Depression
  - Decreased socialization
  - Sleep disturbances
  - Impaired ambulation
  - Increased health care utilization and costs
- Despite the prevalence and impact of pain on older adults, many barriers prevent effective pain assessment and management:
  - Nurse's beliefs that pain is a natural and expected part of aging
  - Older adults' hesitancy to report pain
  - Normal and pathological changes of aging that affect the presentation of pain in older adults
  - The unavailability of objective biological markers of pain
- The most effective method on which nurses must rely to assess pain is the patient's self-report.
- Many standardized tools are available for assessing pain in older adults.
  - A numeric rating scale on which the client is asked to choose a number from 0 to 10 that best describes the pain he or she is experiencing, with 0 being no pain and 10 being the worst pain imaginable

- Visual Analogue Scales (VAS), which are straight horizontal 100-mm lines with verbal pain descriptors on the left and on the right sides.
- The Faces Scale, which depicts six facial expressions on a scale from 0 to 6, with 0 = smile (no pain) and 6 = crying grimace (very much pain). For more information on the Faces Scale, refer to www.iasp-pain.org.

■ Determining the right tool for each patient is necessary to utilize these objective measures effectively. These scales may be used for baseline and subsequent pain assessments to evaluate the effectiveness of treatment. Instruments such as the PAINAD should be used (see Table 11.1).

■ For older adults with cognitive impairments, clients may not be able to verbalize pain appropriately and need special assessment. In these patients, pain behaviors may include:

- Yelling out
- Wandering
- Repetitive behavior
- Aggressive behavior

■ Pain treatment includes:

- Treatment of the underlying cause of pain
- Pharmacological pain management following a "start low and go slow" protocol (American Geriatrics Society, 2009)
  - Acetaminophen
  - Nonsteroidal anti-inflammatory drugs (NSAIDs)
  - Opioids
- Collaborative pain medications, such as
  - Antidepressants
  - Anticonvulsants
  - Anxiolytics
- Nonpharmacological pain management strategies
  - Exercise
  - Educational and cognitive therapy
  - Massage
  - Acupuncture
  - Therapeutic touch
  - Reiki
  - Reflexology

SEXUALITY

■ One of the most prevalent myths of aging is that older adults are no longer interested in sex.

■ A survey of 3,005 U.S. older adults found that sexual activity was reported in 73% of adults age 57 to 64; 53% of adults age 65 to 74; and 26% of adults age 75 to 84 (Lindau et al., 2007).

■ The need to maintain one's sexuality and sexual function should be as highly valued as other physiological needs.

■ Nurses and other health care providers do not regularly assess sexuality, and few intervene to promote the sexuality of the older population because of

• Lack of knowledge

• Lack of education regarding sexuality in aging

• General inexperience and discomfort with the issue

■ The fulfillment of sexual needs may be just as satisfying for older adults as it is for younger people.

TABLE 11.1   Pain Assessment in Advanced Dementia (PAINAD) Scale

ITEMS[a]	0	1	2	SCORE
Breathing independent of vocalization	Normal	Occasional labored breathing	Noisy labored breathing	
		Short period of hyperventilation	Long period of hyperventilation Cheyne–Stokes respirations	
Negative vocalization	None	Occasional moan or groan	Repeated troubled calling out	
		Low-level speech with a negative or disapproving quality	Loud moaning or groaning	
			Crying	
Facial expression	Smiling or inexpressive	Sad Frightened Frown	Facial grimacing	
Body language	Relaxed	Tense Distressed Pacing Fidgeting	Rigid Fists clenched	
			Knees pulled up Pulling or pushing away Striking out	
Consolability	No need to console	Distracted or reassured by voice or touch	Unable to console, distract, or reassure	
				Total[b]

(continued)

TABLE 11.1 Pain Assessment in Advanced Dementia (PAINAD) Scale (*continued*)

Breathing

1. Normal breathing is characterized by effortless, quiet, rhythmic (smooth) respirations.
2. Occasional labored breathing is characterized by episodic bursts of harsh, difficult, or wearing respirations.
3. Short period of hyperventilation is characterized by intervals of rapid, deep breaths lasting a short period of time.
4. Noisy, labored breathing is characterized by negative-sounding respirations on inspiration or expiration. They may be loud, gurgling, or wheezing. They appear strenuous or wearing.
5. Long period of hyperventilation is characterized by an excessive rate and depth of respirations lasting a considerable time.
6. Cheyne–Stokes respirations are characterized by rhythmic waxing and waning of breathing from very deep to shallow respirations with periods of apnea (cessation of breathing).

Negative Vocalization

1. None is characterized by speech or vocalization that has a neutral or pleasant quality.
2. Occasional moan or groan is characterized by mournful or murmuring sounds, wails, or laments. Groaning is characterized by louder-than-usual inarticulate involuntary sounds, often abruptly beginning and ending.
3. Low-level speech with a negative or disapproving quality is characterized by muttering, mumbling, whining, grumbling, or swearing in a low volume with a complaining, sarcastic, or caustic tone.
4. Repeated troubled calling out is characterized by phrases or words being used over and over in a tone that suggests anxiety, uneasiness, or distress.
5. Loud moaning or groaning is characterized by mournful or murmuring sounds, wails, or laments much louder than usual.
   Loud groaning is characterized by louder-than-usual inarticulate involuntary sounds, often abruptly beginning and ending.
6. Crying is characterized by an utterance of emotion accompanied by tears. There may be sobbing or quiet weeping.

Facial Expression

1. Smiling is characterized by upturned corners of the mouth, brightening of the eyes, and a look of pleasure or contentment. Inexpressive refers to a neutral, at ease, relaxed, or blank look.
2. Sad is characterized by an unhappy, lonesome, sorrowful, or dejected look. There may be tears in the eyes.
3. Frightened is characterized by a look of fear, alarm, or heightened anxiety. Eyes appear wide open.
4. Frown is characterized by a downward turn of the corners of the mouth. Increased facial wrinkling in the forehead and around the mouth may appear.
5. Facial grimacing is characterized by a distorted, distressed look. The brow is more wrinkled as is the area around the mouth. Eyes may be squeezed shut.

Body Language

1. Relaxed is characterized by a calm, restful, mellow appearance. The person seems to be taking it easy.
2. Tense is characterized by a strained, apprehensive, or worried appearance. The jaw may be clenched (exclude any contractures).
3. Distressed pacing is characterized by activity that seems unsettled. There may be a fearful, worried, or disturbed element present. The rate may be faster or slower.
4. Fidgeting is characterized by restless movement. Squirming about or wiggling in the chair may occur. The person might be hitching a chair across the room. Repetitive touching, tugging, or rubbing body parts can also be observed.

(*continued*)

TABLE 11.1 Pain Assessment in Advanced Dementia (PAINAD) Scale (*continued*)

5. Rigid is characterized by stiffening of the body. The arms and/or legs are tight and inflexible. The trunk may appear straight and unyielding (exclude any contractures).
6. Clenched fists is characterized by tightly closed hands. They may be opened and closed repeatedly or held tightly shut.
7. Knees pulled up is characterized by flexing the legs and drawing the knees up toward the chest. Presents as an overall troubled appearance (exclude any contractures).
8. Pulling or pushing away is characterized by resistance on approach or to care. The person is trying to escape by yanking or wrenching him or herself free or shoving you away.
9. Striking out is characterized by hitting, kicking, grabbing, punching, biting, or other forms of personal assault.

Consolability

1. No need to console is characterized by a sense of well-being. The person appears content.
2. Distracted or reassured by voice or touch is characterized by a disruption in the behavior when the person is spoken to or touched. The behavior stops during the period of interaction with no indication that the person is at all distressed.
3. Unable to console, distract, or reassure is characterized by the inability to soothe the person or stop a behavior with words or actions. No amount of comforting, verbal or physical, will alleviate the behavior.

Notes: [a] Five-item observational tool (see the description of each item).
[b] Total scores range from 0 to 10 (based on a scale of 0 to 2 for five items), with a higher score indicating more severe pain (0 = no pain to 10 = severe pain).

Reprinted from Warden, Hurley, and Volicer (2003). Copyright 2003, with permission from the American Medical Directors Association.

▧ Sexuality among older adults is complicated by many issues:

● Older adults may experience performance anxiety.

● Older adults may not be familiar with the risks of sexually transmitted diseases and appropriate prevention.

● Negative self-concepts and role changes that frequently occur in response to chronic illness may impact the experience of sexuality for older adults. The results might be

– Fear of rejection or failure

– Boredom

– Hostility about sexual performance

● Past sexual history, such as delays in sexual development or sexual abuse, may continue to impact sexuality in the later years.

● Older adults tend to be reluctant to discuss sexual issues with health care providers.

● Normal physiological changes among aging women:

– A decrease in circulating estrogen, resulting in a thinning of the vaginal epithelium, the labia majora, and the subcutaneous tissue in the mons pubis.

- – The vaginal canal shortens and loses elasticity.
- – Follicular depletion of the ovaries as a result of a decrease in circulating estrogen, which leads to a further decline in the secretion of estrogen and progesterone.
- – Dyspareunia (painful intercourse) may result.
- – Orgasmic dysfunction and vaginismus may also result from the decrease in the amount of circulating estrogen and progesterone.

■ Normal physiological changes among aging men:

- • Viropause, andropause, or male menopause
- • Increased time needed to develop an erection and ejaculate
- • Erections may require direct penile stimulation

■ In both sexes, the physiological changes in hormone secretion affect four areas of sexual response:

- • Arousal
- • Orgasm
- • Postorgasm
- • Extragenital changes

■ Normal changes of aging may change or delay the sexual response of older adults; however, sexual dysfunction is not a normal process of aging.

■ Chronic illnesses, such as depression and diabetes, impact sexual function among older adults.

■ Medications that are commonly used among older adults can affect sexual function. These medications include:

- • Antidepressants
- • Antihypertensives
- • Antipsychotics
- • Statin medications
- • H_2 blockers

■ Surgery to prostate gland and breasts frequently interferes with the normal sexual function of older men and women.

■ The loss of partners in older adulthood also significantly impacts sexuality.

■ A sexual assessment is the first step needed to assess the sexuality of older adults (see Chapter 8 for sexual assessment guidelines).

■ Instruction regarding normal and pathological aging changes is needed.

■ Interventions to promote sexuality among older adults may focus on

- Promotion of erectile function among older men
    - Erectile agents, such as sildenafil citrate (Viagra), vardenafil hydrochloride (Levitra), and tadalafil (Cialis), may aid in the treatment of erectile dysfunction among older men.
    - These medications are hazardous in men with history of heart failure, in patients with borderline hypotension, and with the use of nitrates.
- The use of touch to create intimacy
- Maintenance of privacy for sexual relationships
- Consideration of client safety
    - Necessary equipment, such as grab bars
    - Condoms for safe sex

■ For older adults with dementia, it is essential to conduct highly accurate assessments and document their ability to be involved in the decision-making process.

■ Problematic sexual behaviors may occur in response to unmet sexual needs in older adults with dementia. These may include:

- Public masturbation
- Exposure
- Making sexually inappropriate comments
- Sexual gestures

■ Effective assessment and planning of care can help the older adult to meet his or her sexual needs in a dignified and respectful manner and will likely eliminate the behavior.

TABLE 11.2 The National Institute on Aging Advises Caregivers to Look for the Following Signs of Elder Abuse

---

■ Has trouble sleeping
■ Seems depressed or confused
■ Loses weight for no reason
■ Displays signs of trauma like rocking back and forth
■ Acts agitated or violent
■ Becomes withdrawn
■ Stops taking part in activities enjoyed in the past
■ Has unexplained bruises, burns, or scars on the body
■ Looks messy, with unwashed hair or dirty clothes
■ Develops bed sores or other preventable conditions

From the National Institute of Aging (2014).

ELDER NEGLECT AND ABUSE

▨ It is estimated that approximately one million cases of elder mistreatment occur annually.

▨ This number is likely an underestimation, because elder abuse is frequently not reported for several reasons.

- Victims may fear retaliation.
- Victims may feel shame.
- Victims may have a desire or need to protect the abuser.
- There is a lack of mandatory universal reporting laws.

▨ Elder abuse is difficult to assess (Table 11.2), but red-flag symptoms include:

- Unexplained injuries or signs of neglect or mistreatment
- Mismatch between an older adult's explanation of injury and his or her physical appearance
- Conflicting stories between victim and caregiver
- Caregiver refusal to leave victim alone

▨ Types of abuse:

- Physical abuse—inflicting physical injury or pain
- Emotional or psychological abuse—infliction of mental anguish, such as threats, insults, and purposeful social isolation
- Verbal abuse—the use of negative verbal communication or the withholding of verbal communication for the intentional infliction of emotional distress
- Active neglect—purposeful withholding of necessities
- Passive neglect—caregiver's inability to identify the older adult's needs or to perform the tasks essential to meet the older adult's needs
- Sexual abuse—sexual assault or rape of an older adult
- Financial abuse/misappropriation of property—exploiting the older adult's funds, property, or assets

▨ Many older adults may exhibit characteristics of multiple types of mistreatment with a wide range of severity.

▨ If elder abuse or neglect is suspected, the health care provider must report it immediately to the area ombudsman, whose job it is to act as a clearinghouse for complaints and problems; agency social service personnel; or the local adult protective services.

- Document assessment effectively using photographs when possible.
- Follow through to make sure the older adult is not returned to an unsafe situation.

REFERENCES

American Geriatrics Society Panel on Chronic Pain in Older Persons. (2009). The management of chronic pain in older persons. *Journal of the American Geriatrics Society, 57*, 1331–1346.

Flaherty, E. (2007). *Try this: Pain assessment in older adults*, 7. Retrieved from http://www.hartfordign.org/publications/trythis/issue07.pdf

Lindau, S. T., Schumm, L. P, Laumann, E. O., Levinson, W., O'Muircheartaigh, C. A., & Waite, L. J. (2007). A study of sexuality and health among older adults in the United States. *New England Journal of Medicine, 357*, 762–774.

National Institute of Aging. (2014). *Try this: Pain assessment in older adults*. http://www.nia.nih.gov/health/publication/elder-abuse#how

Pediatric Pain Sourcebook. (2007). *Faces pain scale*. Retrieved March 23, 2008, from http://painsourcebook.ca/pdfs/pps92.pdf

Warden, V., Hurley, A. C., & Volicer, L. (2003). Development and psychometric evaluation of the Pain Assessment in Advanced Dementia (PAINAD) scale. *Journal of the American Medical Directors Association, 4*(1), 9–15.

12

Organizational and Health Policy Issues

ADVOCACY FOR OLDER ADULTS

Older adults as a group have taken action to prevent the effects of ageism on health care policy. Older adults have formed two large and influential national organizations that provide them with representation concerning legislative issues and resources for successful aging.

- AARP
  - AARP is the nation's leading and most powerful organization for people age 50 and older.
  - The organization has substantial influence on policy making at the federal and state levels.
  - AARP has 36 million members—over 50% of older adults.
  - The membership is growing quickly, with a new member joining AARP every 11 seconds.
  - The name is misleading, because many members of AARP are not retired.
  - AARP is a nonprofit, nonpartisan organization whose primary goal is to help older people live with independence, dignity, and purpose.
  - An important component of the organization is its lobbying ability and influence on legislative issues of importance to older adults. With the assistance of AARP, the rights of older adults continue to be heard loudly on Capitol Hill.

- National Council on Aging (NCOA)
  - NCOA is a nonprofit organization that plays an influential role in providing information, technical assistance, and research in the field of aging.
  - It maintains a national information clearinghouse related to aging, plans conferences on aging issues, conducts research on aging, supports demonstration programs related to aging, and maintains a comprehensive

HEALTH CARE DELIVERY SYSTEMS

■ As a result of the vast improvements in health care technology, health care costs increased 12% to 14% per year in the 1970s and began to decrease slightly in the 1980s.

■ Although the health care delivery system has improved vastly over the past century, many of the currently available interventions to detect disease early and treat disease effectively are not accessible to older adults because:

• Many older adults are uninsured.

• Insurance might not cover a necessary test, procedure, or treatment.

• Many older adults lack transportation to health care providers.

• Primary providers of geriatric care are not widely available.

REIMBURSEMENT

■ Reimbursement for health care has changed as a result of increasing costs. Allowable expenses under Medicare and Medicaid plans as well as private insurances have diminished in many cases and have been removed altogether in some cases.

• The lack of reimbursement for medications and treatments for illness and the inability to pay out of pocket for these expensive treatments have resulted in an increase in the rates of noncompliance or nonadherence to medication regimens.

• About half of all patients take the medications as prescribed upon leaving the physician's office. The other half take the medications incorrectly or not at all. One third of those who take the medications incorrectly don't take them at all; one third take some of the medications prescribed; and one third do not even fill the prescription.

• Little, if any, time is spent on how to assist patients without health insurance to obtain needed health care.

• Regardless of the reason, many older adults need financial assistance to pay for health care.

• Hospitals often have programs to help older adults finance their health care over a period of months, or to excuse the older adult from paying if he or she cannot legitimately afford to do so.

• Physicians and other health care providers may offer the same payment alternatives for services received at private physicians' offices.

• Physicians in private practice may also have samples of medications to distribute to low-income older adults.

• Clinics often have sliding scales for fees to make health care in these facilities more affordable. There are also various state-run programs that help older adults with resources for financing or finding health care that is affordable.

OLDER AMERICANS ACT

- Title III of the Older Americans Act of 1965 directed attention toward public and private health care systems to provide improved access to services and advocacy for older adults.

- This program improved community services, such as home-delivered meals, transportation, home health care and homemaking assistance, adult day care, home repair, and legal assistance—all of which allow many older adults to remain functionally independent and community dwelling.

- These programs are administered within local Area Agencies on Aging (AAAs) in each state. AAAs provide older adults and health care providers with a resource with which to access and afford health care.

- To locate the AAA in each state, use the links tab located at www.n4a.org. In addition to this web resource, the Administration on Aging offers a toll-free Eldercare Locator telephone number—(800) 677-1116—to help older adults, families, and health care providers obtain necessary community services throughout the United States. Operators at Eldercare Locator assist callers in finding information and assistance to address health care and other issues to ensure high functioning and quality of life.

- In addition to AAAs, senior service offices in hospitals are good sources of information about hospital and community-based resources.

MEDICARE AND MEDIGAP

- Medicare is a federal program that was enacted into law in 1965 during a time in U.S. history known as the Great Society. Medicare was among several programs that were started during this period with the specific aim of assisting the poor, the disabled, and older people to have a better quality of health care and quality of life.

- Older adults who have not paid into the U.S. Social Security system, either because they were never employed or because they immigrated to the United States as older adults, must buy into the Medicare system to receive these benefits.

- The large majority of people age 65 and older are enrolled in Medicare.

- To be eligible to receive Medicare, older adults must have contributed to Social Security or the Medicare system during their working years or have a spouse who had worked and contributed to these systems.

- Medicare is paid for by the government and therefore involves regulation, including the need for institutions receiving Medicare reimbursement to complete full resident assessment instruments within 14 days and a plan of care within 21 days of facility admission.

- Health care delivery under Medicare is provided by private physicians, hospitals, nurses, nurse practitioners, and various health care facilities, not Medicare employees.

■ Private physicians who treat Medicare patients receive 80% of the usual customary and reasonable (UCR) fee for services provided if they accept Medicare assignment. If they do not, they can charge no more than 115% of the amount allowed by Medicare, and the client must pay the 20% remaining UCR and any other amount up to 115%.

■ Physicians are often hesitant to accept the low reimbursement paid for older adults through Medicare, and patients are hesitant to receive care from physicians who do not accept Medicare assignment because of the need to finance the co-pay. Consequently, there is a shortage of primary care physicians available to treat the increasing health care needs of older adults.

■ Medicare has two parts:

- Part A provides hospital insurance for older adults. In the event that an older adult requires hospitalization, this is the type of Medicare insurance that would pay for the hospital stay. In addition, this is the portion of Medicare that pays for short-term nursing home or home care visits after hospitalization in order for the older adult to return to prehospitalization health status. Medicare Part A also pays for hospice care (discussed in Chapter 7). Generally, there is no premium for this insurance. In other words, if older adults meet the eligibility for Medicare as previously stated, they are automatically enrolled in the Part A Medicare plan.

- Part B pays for visits to physicians, nurse practitioners, and for other health care expenditures, such as x-rays, physical and occupational outpatient therapy, and laboratory tests. There is a monthly premium that older adults must pay for this type of Medicare plan. The current monthly premium is about $140.90. The amount is usually deducted from the recipient's monthly Social Security checks. Part B Medicare also requires recipients to pay the first $147 of charges before it will begin reimbursement. This is known as a deductible. The deductible for Part B Medicare is likely to increase annually. Coverage of Medicare for health care needs of older adults is detailed in Table 12.1.

■ The Medicare traditional plan previously described has undergone much scrutiny since its inception in 1965. From a government perspective, providing Medicare coverage to an increasingly larger cohort of older adults is challenging and has resulted in limited reimbursement to health care professionals. Attempts to resolve some of these issues, numerous changes, and additions to the traditional Medicare plan have evolved.

■ Medigap is private (nongovernmental) health insurance available to Medicare recipients for purchase to help pay for what Medicare does not cover.

■ Some of the health care expenses covered by Medigap include Medicare deductibles, co-pays (the additional amount of money that the patient must pay the health care provider), health care outside the United States, and medications.

■ The federal government has set regulations that must be followed by the providers of these plans.

TABLE 12.1   Medicare Coverage for the Health Care Needs of Older Adults

SERVICE OR SUPPLY	What is covered, and when?
Acupuncture	Medicare doesn't cover acupuncture.
Ambulance Services	Medicare covers limited ambulance services. If you need to go to a hospital or skilled nursing facility (SNF), ambulance services are covered only if transportation in any other vehicle would endanger your health. Medicare helps pay for necessary ambulance transportation to the closest appropriate facility that can provide the care you need. If you choose to go to another facility farther away, Medicare payment is 80% of how much it should cost to go to the closest appropriate facility. All ambulance suppliers must accept the assignment. Medicare generally doesn't pay for ambulance transportation to a doctor's office. Air ambulance is paid only in the most severe situations. If you could have gone by land ambulance without serious danger to your life or health, Medicare pays only the land ambulance rate, and you are responsible for the difference.
Ambulatory Surgical Centers	Medicare covers 80% of the cost of services given in an ambulatory surgical center for a covered surgical procedure.
Anesthesia	Medicare covers 80% of the approved amount for anesthesia services along with medical and surgical benefits. Medicare Part A covers anesthesia you get while in an inpatient hospital. Medicare Part B covers anesthesia you get as an outpatient.
Artificial Limbs and Eyes	Medicare helps pay for artificial limbs and eyes. For more information, see Prosthetic Devices.
Blood	Medicare doesn't cover the first three pints of blood you get under Part A and B combined in a calendar year. Part A covers blood you get as an inpatient, and Part B covers blood you get as an outpatient and in a freestanding Ambulatory Surgical Center.
Bone Mass Measurement	Medicare covers bone mass measurements ordered by a doctor or qualified practitioner who is treating you if you meet one or more of the following conditions: Women ▧ You are being treated for low estrogen levels and are at clinical risk for osteoporosis, based on your medical history and other findings. Men and Women ▧ Your x-rays show possible osteoporosis, osteopenia, or vertebrae fractures. ▧ You are on prednisone or steroid-type drugs or are planning to begin such treatment. ▧ You have been diagnosed with primary hyperparathyroidism. ▧ You are being monitored to see if your osteoporosis drug therapy is working. The test is covered once every 2 years for qualified individuals and more often if medically necessary.
Braces (arm, leg, back, and neck)	Medicare covers 80% of the approved amount for arm, leg, back, and neck braces. For more information, see Orthotics.
Breast Prostheses	Medicare covers breast prostheses (including a surgical brassiere) after a mastectomy. For more information, see Prosthetic Devices.

TABLE 12.1   Medicare Coverage for the Health Care Needs of Older Adults (*continued*)

Canes/Crutches	Medicare covers 80% of the approved amount for canes and crutches. Medicare doesn't cover canes for the blind. For more information, see Durable Medical Equipment (DME).
Cardiac Rehabilitation Programs	Medicare covers 80% of the approved amount for comprehensive programs that include exercise, education, and counseling for patients whose doctor referred them and who have (1) had a heart attack in the past 12 months, (2) had coronary bypass surgery, (3) stable angina pectoris, (4) had heart valve repair/replacement, (5) had angioplasty or coronary stenting, and/or (6) had a heart or heart–lung transplant. These programs may be given by the outpatient department of a hospital or in doctor-directed clinics.
Cardiovascular Screening	Medicare covers screening tests for cholesterol, lipid, and triglyceride levels every 5 years. Ask your doctor to test your cholesterol, lipid, and triglyceride levels so he or she can help you prevent a heart attack or stroke.
Chemotherapy	Medicare covers 80% of the approved amount for chemotherapy for patients who are hospital inpatients, outpatients, or patients in a doctor's office or freestanding clinics. In the inpatient hospital setting, Part A covers chemotherapy. However, in a hospital outpatient setting, freestanding facility, or doctor's office, Part B covers chemotherapy.
Chiropractic Services	Medicare covers 80% of the approved costs of manipulation of the spine if medically necessary to correct a subluxation (when one or more of the bones of your spine moves out of position) when provided by chiropractors or other qualified providers.
Clinical Trials	Medicare covers 80% of routine costs, such as doctor visits and tests, if you take part in a qualifying clinical trial. Clinical trials test new types of medical care, like how well a new cancer drug works. Clinical trials help doctors and researchers see if the new care works and if it is safe. Medicare doesn't pay for the experimental item being investigated, in most cases.
Colorectal Cancer Screening	Medicare covers several colorectal cancer screening tests. Talk with your doctor about the screening test that is right for you. All people age 50 and older with Medicare are covered. However, there is no minimum age for having a colonoscopy. Colonoscopy: Medicare covers 80% of the approved cost of this test once every 24 months if you are at high risk for colorectal cancer. If you aren't at high risk for colorectal cancer, the test is covered once every 120 months, but not sooner than 48 months after a screening sigmoidoscopy. Fecal Occult Blood Test: Medicare covers this lab test once every 12 months. Flexible Sigmoidoscopy: Medicare covers this test once every 48 months for people 50 and older. Barium Enema: Once every 48 months (high risk every 24 months) when used instead of a flexible sigmoidoscopy or colonoscopy.
Commode Chairs	Medicare covers 80% of the approved cost of commode chairs that your doctor orders for use in your home if you are confined to your bedroom. For more information, see DME.

(*continued*)

TABLE 12.1   Medicare Coverage for the Health Care Needs of Older Adults (*continued*)

Cosmetic Surgery	Medicare generally doesn't cover cosmetic surgery unless it is needed because of accidental injury or to improve the function of a malformed part of the body. Medicare covers breast reconstruction if you had a mastectomy because of breast cancer.
Custodial Care (help with activities of daily living, like bathing, dressing, using the bathroom, and eating)	Medicare doesn't cover custodial care when it's the only kind of care you need. Care is considered custodial when it's for the purpose of helping you with activities of daily living or personal needs that could be done safely and reasonably by people without professional skills or training. For example, custodial care includes help getting in and out of bed, bathing, dressing, eating, and taking medicine.
Dental Services	Medicare doesn't cover routine dental care or most dental procedures, such as cleanings, fillings, tooth extractions, or dentures. Medicare doesn't pay for dental plates or other dental devices. Medicare Part A will pay for certain dental services that you get when you are in the hospital. Medicare Part A can pay for hospital stays if you need to have emergency or complicated dental procedures, even when the dental care itself isn't covered.
Diabetes Screening	Medicare covers tests to check for diabetes. These tests are available if you have any of the following risk factors: high blood pressure, dyslipidemia (history of abnormal cholesterol and triglyceride levels), obesity, or a history of high blood sugar. Medicare also covers these tests if you have two or more of the following characteristics: ■ age 65 or older ■ overweight ■ family history of diabetes (parents, brothers, and sisters) ■ a history of gestational diabetes (diabetes during pregnancy) or delivery of a baby weighing more than 9 pounds Based on the results of these tests, you may be eligible for up to two diabetes screenings every year.
Diabetes Supplies and Services	Medicare covers some diabetes supplies, including ■ blood glucose test strips ■ blood glucose monitor ■ lancet devices and lancets ■ glucose control solutions for checking the accuracy of test strips and monitors There may be limits on how much or how often you get these supplies. For more information, see DME. Here are some ways you can make sure your Medicare diabetes medical supplies are covered: ■ Only accept supplies you have ordered. Medicare won't pay for supplies you didn't order. ■ Make sure you request your supply refills. Medicare won't pay for supplies sent from the supplier to you automatically. ■ All Medicare-enrolled pharmacies and suppliers must submit claims for glucose test strips. You can't send in the claim yourself. Medicare doesn't cover insulin (unless used with an insulin pump), insulin pens, syringes, needles, alcohol swabs, gauze, eye exams for

---

(continued)

TABLE 12.1   Medicare Coverage for the Health Care Needs of Older Adults (*continued*)

---

glasses, and routine or yearly physical exams. If you use an external insulin pump, insulin and the pump could be covered as DME.

There may be some limits on covered supplies or how often you get them. Insulin and certain medical supplies used to inject insulin are covered under Medicare prescription drug coverage.

Therapeutic Shoes or Inserts: Medicare covers 80% of the approved cost of therapeutic shoes or inserts for people with diabetes who have severe diabetic foot disease. The doctor who treats your diabetes must certify your need for therapeutic shoes or inserts. The shoes and inserts must be prescribed by a podiatrist or other qualified doctor and provided by a podiatrist, orthotist, prosthetist, or pedorthist. Medicare helps pay for one pair of therapeutic shoes and inserts per calendar year. Shoe modifications may be substituted for inserts. The fitting of the shoes or inserts is covered in the Medicare payment for the shoes.

Medicare covers these diabetes services:

■ Diabetes Self-Management Training: Diabetes outpatient self-management training is a covered program to teach you to manage your diabetes. It includes education about self-monitoring of blood glucose, diet, exercise, and insulin.

If you've been diagnosed with diabetes, Medicare may cover 80% of the approved cost for up to 10 hours of initial diabetes self-management training.

You may also qualify for up to 2 hours of follow-up training each year if

■ it is provided in a group of 2 to 20 people
■ it lasts for at least 30 minutes
■ it takes place in a calendar year following the year you got your initial training
■ your doctor or a qualified nonphysician practitioner ordered it as part of your plan of care

Some exceptions apply if no group session is available or if your doctor or qualified nonphysician practitioner says you have special needs that prevent you from participating in group training.

Yearly Eye Exam: Medicare covers 80% of the cost of yearly eye exams for diabetic retinopathy.

Foot Exam: 80% of the approved cost of a foot exam is covered every 6 months for people with diabetic peripheral neuropathy and loss of protective sensations, as long as you haven't seen a foot care professional for another reason between visits.

Glaucoma Screening: Medicare covers glaucoma screening every 12 months for people with diabetes or a family history of glaucoma, African Americans age 50 and older, or Hispanics age 65 and older.

Medical Nutrition Therapy Services: Medical nutrition therapy services are also covered for people with diabetes or kidney disease when referred by a doctor. These services can be given by a registered dietitian or Medicare-approved nutrition professional and include a nutritional assessment and counseling to help you manage your diabetes or kidney disease.

For more information, call 1-800-MEDICARE (1-800-633-4227). TTY users should call 1-877-486-2048.

(*continued*)

TABLE 12.1   Medicare Coverage for the Health Care Needs of Older Adults (*continued*)

Diagnostic Tests, X-rays, and Lab Services	Medicare covers 80% of approved costs for diagnostic tests like CT scans, MRIs, EKGs, and x-rays. Medicare also covers clinical diagnostic tests and lab services provided by certified laboratories enrolled in Medicare. Diagnostic tests and lab services are done to help your doctor diagnose or rule out a suspected illness or condition. Medicare doesn't cover most routine screening tests, like checking your hearing. Some preventive tests and screenings are covered by Medicare to help prevent, find, or manage a medical problem. For more information, see Preventive Services.
Dialysis (Kidney)	Medicare covers 80% of the approved amount of some kidney dialysis services and supplies, including the following: ■ Inpatient dialysis treatments (if you are admitted to a hospital for special care) ■ Outpatient maintenance dialysis treatments (when you get treatments in any Medicare-approved dialysis facility) ■ Certain home dialysis support services (may include visits by trained dialysis workers to check on your home dialysis, to help in dialysis emergencies when needed, and check your dialysis equipment and hemodialysis water supply) ■ Certain drugs for home dialysis, including heparin, the antidote for heparin when medically necessary, and topical anesthetics ■ Erythropoiesis–stimulating agents (such as Epogen, epoetin alfa), or darbepoetin alfa (Aranesp) are drugs used to treat anemia if you have end-stage renal disease; for more information, see Prescription Drugs ■ Self-dialysis training (includes training for you and the person helping you with your home dialysis treatments) ■ Home dialysis equipment and supplies (i.e., alcohol, wipes, sterile drapes, rubber gloves, and scissors)
Doctor's Office Visits	Medicare covers 80% of the approved cost of medically necessary services you get from your doctor in his or her office, in a hospital, in an SNF, in your home, or any other location. Routine annual physicals aren't covered, except the one-time "Welcome to Medicare" physical exam. Some preventive tests and screenings are covered by Medicare. See Preventive Services and Pap Test/Pelvic Exam.
Drugs	See Prescription Drugs (Outpatient).
DME	Medicare covers 80% of the approved cost of DME that your doctor prescribes for use in your home. Only your own doctor can prescribe medical equipment for you. DME is ■ (long lasting) durable ■ used for a medical reason ■ not usually useful to someone who isn't sick or injured ■ used in your home The DME that Medicare covers includes, but isn't limited to, the following: ■ Air-fluidized beds ■ Blood glucose monitors ■ Canes (canes for the blind aren't covered)

(continued)

TABLE 12.1 Medicare Coverage for the Health Care Needs of Older Adults (*continued*)

	■ Commode chairs ■ Crutches ■ Dialysis machines ■ Home oxygen equipment and supplies ■ Hospital beds ■ Infusion pumps (and some medicines used in infusion pumps if considered reasonable and necessary) ■ Nebulizers (and some medicines used in nebulizers if considered reasonable and necessary) ■ Patient lifts (to lift patient from bed or wheelchair by hydraulic operation) ■ Suction pumps ■ Traction equipment ■ Walkers ■ Wheelchairs Make sure your supplier is enrolled in Medicare and has a Medicare supplier number. Suppliers have to meet strict standards to qualify for a Medicare supplier number. Medicare won't pay your claim if your supplier doesn't have one, even if your supplier is a large chain or department store that sells more than just DME.
Emergency Room Services	Medicare covers 80% of the approved cost of emergency room services, after the deductible. Emergency services aren't covered in foreign countries, except in some instances in Canada and Mexico. For more information, see Travel. A medical emergency is when you believe that your health is in serious danger. You may have an injury or illness that requires immediate medical attention to prevent a severe disability or death. When you go to an emergency room, you will pay a copayment for each hospital service, and you will also pay coinsurance for each doctor who treats you. *Note:* If you are admitted to the hospital within 3 days of the emergency room visit for the same condition, the emergency room visit is included in the inpatient hospital care charges, not charged separately.
Equipment	See DME.
Eye Exams	Medicare doesn't cover routine eye exams. Medicare covers some preventive eye tests and screenings: ■ See yearly eye exams under Diabetes Supplies and Services ■ See Glaucoma Screening ■ See Macular Degeneration
Eyeglasses/Contact Lenses	Generally, Medicare doesn't cover eyeglasses or contact lenses. However, following cataract surgery with an implanted intraocular lens, Medicare helps pay for corrective lenses (spectacles or contact lenses) provided by a licensed and Medicare-approved ophthalmologist. Services provided by a licensed and Medicare-approved ophthalmologist may be covered, if they are authorized to provide this service in your state. Important: ■ Only standard frames are covered. ■ Lenses are covered even if you had the surgery before you had Medicare. ■ Payment may be made for lenses for both eyes even though cataract surgery involved only one eye.

(continued)

TABLE 12.1   Medicare Coverage for the Health Care Needs of Older Adults (*continued*)

Eye Refractions	Medicare doesn't cover eye refractions.
Flu Shots	Medicare covers one flu shot per flu season. You can get a flu shot in the winter and the fall flu season of the same calendar year. All people with Medicare are covered.
Foot Care	Medicare generally doesn't cover routine foot care. Medicare Part B covers the 80% of the approved cost of the services of a podiatrist (foot doctor) for medically necessary treatment of injuries or diseases of the foot (i.e., hammer toe, bunion deformities, and heel spurs). 　　See Therapeutic Shoes or Inserts and Foot Exam under Diabetes Supplies and Services.
Glaucoma Screening	Medicare covers 80% of the approved cost of glaucoma screening once every 12 months for people at high risk for glaucoma. This includes people with diabetes, a family history of glaucoma, African Americans age 50 and older, or Hispanic Americans age 65 and older. The screening must be done or supervised by an eye doctor who is legally allowed to do this service in your state.
Health Education/ Wellness Programs	Medicare generally doesn't cover health education and wellness programs. However, Medicare does cover medical nutrition therapy for some people and diabetes education for people with diabetes.
Hearing Exams/ Hearing Aids	Medicare doesn't cover routine hearing exams, hearing aids, or exams for fitting hearing aids. In some cases, Medicare covers diagnostic hearing exams.
Hepatitis B Shots	Medicare covers this preventive service (three shots) for people at high or medium (intermediate) to high risk for hepatitis B. 　　Your risk for hepatitis B increases if you have hemophilia, end-stage renal disease (permanent kidney failure requiring dialysis or a kidney transplant), or a condition that lowers your resistance to infection. Other factors may also increase your risk for hepatitis B. Check with your doctor to see if you are at high to medium risk for hepatitis B.
Home Health Care	Medicare covers some home health care if the following conditions are met: 1. Your doctor decides you need medical care in your home and makes a plan for your care at home. 2. You need reasonable and necessary part-time or intermittent skilled nursing care and home health aide services, and physical therapy, occupational therapy, and speech–language pathology ordered by your doctor and provided by a Medicare-certified home health agency. This includes medical social services, other services, DME (i.e., wheelchairs, hospital beds, oxygen, and walkers), and medical supplies for use at home. 3. You are homebound. This means you are normally unable to leave home and that leaving home is a major effort. When you leave home, it must be infrequent, for a short time. You may attend religious services. You may leave the house to get medical treatment, including therapeutic or psychosocial care. You can also get care in an adult day care program that is licensed or certified by your state or accredited to furnish adult day care services in your state. 4. The home health agency caring for you must be approved by Medicare.

TABLE 12.1 Medicare Coverage for the Health Care Needs of Older Adults (*continued*)

	Medicare covers DME (i.e., wheelchairs, hospital beds, oxygen, and walkers). *Note for Women With Osteoporosis*: Medicare helps pay 80% of the approved amount for an injectable drug for osteoporosis in women who have Medicare Part B, meet the criteria for the Medicare home health benefit, and have a bone fracture that a doctor certifies was related to postmenopausal osteoporosis. You must also be certified by a doctor as unable to learn or unable to give yourself the drug by injection, and that family and/or caregivers are unable or unwilling to give the drug by injection. Medicare covers the visit by a home health nurse to give the drug.

Hospice Care	Medicare covers hospice care if
	▣ you are eligible for Medicare Part A
	▣ your doctor and the hospice medical director certify that you are terminally ill and probably have less than 6 months to live
	▣ you accept palliative (care to comfort) instead of care to cure your illness
	▣ you sign a statement choosing hospice care instead of routine Medicare-covered benefits for your terminal illness
	▣ you get care from a Medicare-approved hospice program
	
	Medicare allows a nurse practitioner to serve as an attending doctor for a patient who elects the hospice benefit.
	    Nurse practitioners are prohibited from certifying a terminal diagnosis.
	    Respite Care: Medicare also covers a portion of the cost of respite care if you are getting covered hospice care. Respite care is inpatient care given to a hospice patient so that the usual caregiver can rest. You can stay in a Medicare-approved facility, such as a hospice facility, hospital or nursing home, up to 5 days each time you get respite care.
	    Medicare will still pay for covered services for any health problems that aren't related to your terminal illness.

Hospital Bed	See DME.
Hospital Care (Inpatient) for Outpatient Services	Medicare covers inpatient hospital care when all of the following are true: ▣ A doctor says you need inpatient hospital care to treat your illness or injury. ▣ You need the kind of care that can be given only in a hospital. ▣ The hospital is enrolled in Medicare. ▣ The Utilization Review Committee of the hospital approves your stay while you are in the hospital. ▣ A quality improvement organization approves your stay after the bill is submitted. Medicare-covered hospital services include the following: a semiprivate room, meals, general nursing, and other hospital services and supplies. This includes care you get in critical access hospitals and inpatient mental health care. This doesn't include private-duty nursing, a television, or telephone in your room. It also doesn't include a private room, unless medically necessary. The cost of the deductibles for hospital inpatient care can be substantial, and the costs vary depending on the duration of the hospital stay.
Implantable Cardiac Defibrillator	Medicare covers defibrillators for many people diagnosed with congestive heart failure.

TABLE 12.1 Medicare Coverage for the Health Care Needs of Older Adults (*continued*)

Kidney (Dialysis)	See Dialysis.
Lab Services	Medicare covers medically necessary diagnostic lab services that are ordered by your treating doctor when they are provided by a Clinical Laboratory Improvement Amendments (CLIA)–certified laboratory enrolled in Medicare. For more information, see Diagnostic Tests.
Macular Degeneration	Medicare covers 80% of the approved cost of certain treatments for some patients with age-related macular degeneration (AMD) like ocular photodynamic therapy with verteporfin (Visudyne).
Mammogram (Screening)	Medicare covers a screening mammogram once every 12 months (11 full months must have gone by from the last screening) for all women with Medicare age 40 and older. You can also get one baseline mammogram between ages 35 and 39.
Mental Health Care	Medicare covers mental health care given by a doctor or a qualified mental health professional. Before you get treatment, ask your doctor, psychologist, social worker, or other health professional if they accept Medicare payment. Inpatient Mental Health Care: Medicare covers inpatient mental health care services. These services can be given in psychiatric units of a general hospital or in a specialty psychiatric hospital that cares for people with mental health problems. Medicare helps pay for inpatient mental health services in the same way that it pays for all other inpatient hospital care. *Note*: If you are in a specialty psychiatric hospital, Medicare only helps for a total of 190 days of inpatient care during your lifetime. Outpatient Mental Health Care: Medicare covers mental health services on an outpatient basis by either a doctor, clinical psychologist, clinical social worker, clinical nurse specialist, or physician assistant in an office setting, clinic, or hospital outpatient department. Partial Hospitalization: Partial hospitalization may be available for you. It is a structured program of active psychiatric treatment that is more intense than the care you get in your doctor or therapist's office. For Medicare to cover a partial hospitalization program, a doctor must say that you would otherwise need inpatient treatment. Medicare covers the services of specially qualified nonphysician practitioners, such as clinical psychologists, clinical social workers, nurse practitioners, clinical nurse specialists, and physician assistants, as allowed by state and local law for medically necessary services.
Nursing Home Care	Most nursing home care is custodial care. Generally, Medicare doesn't cover custodial care. Medicare Part A only covers skilled nursing care given in a certified SNF or in your home (if you are homebound) if medically necessary, but not custodial care (i.e., helping with bathing or dressing).
Nutrition Therapy Services (Medical)	Medicare covers medical nutrition therapy services, when ordered by a doctor, for people with kidney disease (but who aren't on dialysis) or who have a kidney transplant, or people with diabetes. These services can be given by a registered dietitian or Medicare-approved nutrition professional and include nutritional assessment, one-on-one counseling, and

(*continued*)

TABLE 12.1   Medicare Coverage for the Health Care Needs of Older Adults (*continued*)

	therapy through an interactive telecommunications system. See Diabetes Supplies and Services.
Occupational Therapy	See Physical Therapy/Occupational Therapy/Speech–Language Pathology.
Orthotics	Medicare covers artificial limbs and eyes; and arm, leg, back, and neck braces. Medicare doesn't pay for orthopedic shoes unless they are a necessary part of the leg brace. Medicare doesn't pay for dental plates or other dental devices. See Diabetes Supplies and Services (Therapeutic Shoes).
Ostomy Supplies	Medicare covers 80% of the approved cost for ostomy supplies for people who have had a colostomy, ileostomy, or urinary ostomy. Medicare covers the amount of supplies your doctor says you need, based on your condition.
Outpatient Hospital Services	Medicare covers medically necessary services you get as an outpatient from a Medicare-participating hospital for diagnosis or treatment of an illness or injury. Medicare generally pays 80% of the approved amount for these services. Covered outpatient hospital services include ■ services in an emergency room or outpatient clinic, including same-day surgery ■ laboratory tests billed by the hospital ■ mental health care in a partial hospitalization program, if a doctor certifies that inpatient treatment would be required without it ■ x-rays and other radiology services billed by the hospitals ■ medical supplies such as splints and casts ■ screenings and preventive services ■ certain drugs and biologicals that you can't give yourself
Oxygen Therapy	Medicare covers 80% of the approved amount of the rental of oxygen equipment. Or, if you own your own equipment, Medicare will help pay for oxygen contents and supplies for the delivery of oxygen when all of these conditions are met: ■ Your doctor says you have a severe lung disease or you're not getting enough oxygen and your condition might improve with oxygen therapy. ■ Your arterial blood gas level falls within a certain range. ■ Other alternative measures have failed. Under these conditions Medicare helps pay for ■ systems for furnishing oxygen ■ containers that store oxygen ■ tubing and related supplies for the delivery of oxygen ■ oxygen contents If oxygen is provided only for use during sleep, portable oxygen wouldn't be covered. Portable oxygen isn't covered when provided only as a backup to a stationary oxygen system.
Pap Test/Pelvic Exam	Medicare covers 80% of the approved cost for Pap tests and pelvic exams (and a clinical breast exam) for all women once every 24 months. Medicare covers this test and exam once every 12 months if you are at high risk for cervical or vaginal cancer or if you are of childbearing age and have had an abnormal Pap test in the past 36 months. If you have your Pap test, pelvic exam, and clinical breast exam on the same visit as a routine

---

TABLE 12.1   Medicare Coverage for the Health Care Needs of Older Adults (*continued*)

---

	physical exam, you pay for the physical exam. Routine physical exams aren't covered by Medicare, except for the one-time "Welcome to Medicare" physical exam.
Physical Exams (routine) (one-time "Welcome to Medicare" physical exam)	Routine physical exams aren't generally covered by Medicare. Medicare covers a one-time review of your health (termed a "wellness check"), as well as education and counseling about the preventive services you need, including certain screenings and shots. Referrals for other care, if you need them, will also be covered. *Important*: You must have the physical exam within the first 6 months you have Medicare Part B (deductibles and coinsurance apply).
Physical Therapy/ Occupational Therapy/Speech– Language Pathology	Medicare helps pay for medically necessary outpatient physical and occupational therapy and speech–language pathology services when ■ your doctor or therapist sets up the plan of treatment ■ your doctor periodically reviews the plan to see how long you will need therapy. You can get outpatient services from a Medicare-approved outpatient provider such as a participating hospital or SNF, or from a participating home health agency, rehabilitation agency, or a comprehensive outpatient rehabilitation facility. Also, you can get services from a Medicare-approved physical or occupational therapist, in private practice, in his or her office, or in your home. (Medicare doesn't pay for services given by a speech–language pathologist in private practice.) There are caps on physical therapy, occupational therapy, and speech–language pathology services. If so, there may be exceptions to these limits.
Pneumococcal Shot	Medicare covers the pneumococcal shot to help prevent pneumococcal infections. Most people only need this preventive shot once in their lifetime. Talk with your doctor to see if you need this shot.
Prescription Drugs (Outpatient) Very Limited Coverage	Part B covers a limited number of outpatient prescription drugs. Your pharmacy or doctor must accept assignment on Medicare-covered prescription drugs. Part B covers drugs that aren't usually self-administered when you are given them in a hospital outpatient department. You can get comprehensive drug coverage by joining a Medicare drug plan (also called "Part D"). The following outpatient prescription drugs are covered: ■ Some Antigens: Medicare will help pay for antigens if they are prepared by a doctor and given by a properly instructed person (who could be the patient) under doctor supervision. ■ Osteoporosis Drugs: Medicare helps pay for an injectable drug for osteoporosis for certain women with Medicare. See note for women with osteoporosis, under Home Health Care. ■ Erythropoiesis-stimulating agents (such as Epogen, Epoetin alfa, or Darbepoetin alfa Aranesp): Medicare will help pay for erythropoietin by injection if you have end-stage renal disease (permanent kidney failure) and need this drug to treat anemia.

(continued)

TABLE 12.1   Medicare Coverage for the Health Care Needs of Older Adults (*continued*)

	■ Blood Clotting Factors: If you have hemophilia, Medicare will help pay for clotting factors you give yourself by injection.
	■ Injectable Drugs: Medicare covers most injectable drugs given by a licensed medical practitioner, if the drug is considered reasonable and necessary for treatment.
	■ Immunosuppressive Drugs: Medicare covers immunosuppressive drug therapy for transplant patients if the transplant was paid for by Medicare (or paid by private insurance that paid as a primary payer to your Medicare Part A coverage) in a Medicare-certified facility.
	■ Oral Cancer Drugs: Medicare will help pay for some cancer drugs you take by mouth if the same drug is available in injectable form.
	Currently, Medicare covers the following cancer drugs you take by mouth:
	• Capecitabine (brand name Xeloda) • Cyclophosphamide (brand name Cytoxan) • Methotrexate • Temozolomide (brand name Temodar) • Busulfan (brand name Myleran) • Etoposide (brand name VePesid) • Melphalan (brand name Alkeran)
	As new cancer drugs become available, Medicare may cover them.
	■ Oral Anti-Nausea Drugs: Medicare will help pay for oral antinausea drugs used as part of an anticancer chemotherapeutic regimen. The drugs must be administered within 48 hours and must be used as a full therapeutic replacement for the intravenous antinausea drugs that would otherwise be given.
	Medicare also covers some drugs used in infusion pumps and nebulizers if considered reasonable and necessary.
Preventive Services	Medicare covers the following preventive services:
	■ Bone mass measurement ■ Cardiovascular screening blood tests ■ Colorectal cancer screening ■ Diabetes screenings ■ Glaucoma screening ■ Mammogram screening ■ Nutrition therapy services ■ Pap test/pelvic exam ■ Prostate cancer screening ■ Shots including
	• flu shot • pneumococcal shot • Hepatitis B shot
	■ Smoking cessation counseling ■ One-time "Welcome to Medicare" physical exam
Prostate Cancer Screening	Medicare covers 80% of the approved amount for prostate screening tests once every 12 months for all men age 50 and older with Medicare (coverage begins the day after your 50th birthday). Covered tests include the following:

(continued)

TABLE 12.1   Medicare Coverage for the Health Care Needs of Older Adults (*continued*)

	■ Digital rectal examination (covered at 80%) ■ Prostate-specific antigen (PSA) test (no cost)
Prosthetic Devices	Medicare covers prosthetic devices needed to replace an internal body part or function. These include Medicare-approved corrective lenses needed after a cataract operation (see Eyeglasses/Contact Lenses), ostomy bags and certain related supplies (see Ostomy Supplies), and breast prostheses (including a surgical brassiere) after a mastectomy (see Breast Prostheses).
Radiation Therapy	Medicare covers 80% of the approved amount for radiation therapy for patients who are hospital inpatients or outpatients or patients in freestanding clinics.
Religious Nonmedical Health Care Institution (RNHCI)	Medicare doesn't cover the religious portion of RNHCI care. Medicare covers inpatient nonmedical care when the following conditions are met: ■ The RNHCI has agreed and is currently certified to participate in Medicare, and the Utilization Review Committee agrees that you'd require hospital or SNF care if it weren't for your religious beliefs. ■ You have a written agreement with Medicare indicating that your need for this form of care is based on your religious beliefs. The agreement must also indicate that if you decide to accept standard medical care you may have to wait longer to get RNHCI services in the future. You're always able to access medically necessary Medicare Part A services. ■ The care provided is reasonable and necessary.
Respite Care	Medicare covers 95% of the cost of respite care for hospice patients (see Hospice Care).
Second Surgical Opinions	Medicare covers a second opinion before surgery that isn't an emergency. A second opinion is when another doctor gives his or her view about your health problem and how it should be treated. Medicare will also help pay for a third opinion if the first and second opinions are different.
Shots (Vaccinations)	Medicare covers the following shots: Flu Shot: Once per flu season. You can get a flu shot in the fall and the winter flu seasons of the same year. Hepatitis B Shot: Certain people with Medicare at medium to high risk for hepatitis B. Pneumococcal Shot: One shot may be all you ever need. Ask your doctor.
SNF Care	Medicare covers skilled care in an SNF under certain conditions for a limited time. Skilled care is health care given when you need skilled nursing or rehabilitation staff to manage, observe, and evaluate your care. Examples of skilled care include changing sterile dressings and physical therapy. Care that can be given by nonprofessional staff isn't considered skilled care. Medicare covers certain skilled care services that are needed daily on a short-term basis (up to 100 days). Medicare will cover skilled care if all these conditions are met: 1. You have Medicare Part A (Hospital Insurance) and have days left in your benefit period to use.

(*continued*)

TABLE 12.1   Medicare Coverage for the Health Care Needs of Older Adults (*continued*)

---

2. You have a qualifying hospital stay. This means an inpatient hospital stay of 3 consecutive days or more, including the day you're admitted to the hospital, but not including the day you leave the hospital. You must enter the SNF within a short time (generally 30 days) of leaving the hospital and require skilled services related to your hospital stay (see item 5). After you leave the SNF, if you reenter the same or another SNF within 30 days, you don't need another 3-day qualifying hospital stay to get additional SNF benefits. This is also true if you stop getting skilled care while in the SNF and then start getting skilled care again within 30 days.
3. Your doctor has decided that you need daily skilled care. It must be given by, or under the direct supervision of, skilled nursing or rehabilitation staff. If you are in the SNF for skilled rehabilitation services only, your care is considered daily care even if these therapy services are offered just 5 or 6 days a week, as long as you need and get the therapy services each day they are offered.
4. You get these skilled services in an SNF that is certified by Medicare.
5. You need these skilled services for a medical condition that
   ■ was treated during a qualifying 3-day hospital stay, or
   ■ started while you were getting care in the SNF for a medical condition that was treated during a qualifying 3-day hospital stay. For example, if you are in the SNF because you had a stroke, and you develop an infection that requires IV antibiotics and you meet the conditions listed in items 1 to 4, Medicare will cover skilled care.

Smoking Cessation (Counseling to Stop Smoking)	Medicare covers minimal regular doctor's office visits, and up to eight face-to-face visits in a 12-month period if you are diagnosed with an illness caused or complicated by tobacco use, or you take a medicine that is affected by tobacco.
Speech–Language Pathology	See Physical Therapy/Occupational Therapy/Speech–Language Pathology.
Substance-Related Disorders	Medicare covers treatment for substance-related disorders in inpatient or outpatient settings. Certain limits apply.
Supplies (You Use at Home)	Medicare generally doesn't cover common medical supplies like bandages and gauze. Supplies furnished as part of a doctor's service are covered by Medicare, and payment is included in Medicare's doctor payment. Doctors don't bill for supplies. Medicare covers some diabetes and dialysis supplies. See Diabetes Supplies and Services and Dialysis (Kidney). For items such as walkers, oxygen, and wheelchairs, see DME.
Surgical Dressings	Medicare covers surgical dressings when medically necessary for the treatment of a surgical or surgically treated wound.
Therapeutic Shoes	See Diabetes Supplies and Services (Therapeutic Shoes).
Transplants (Doctor Services)	Medicare covers doctor services for transplants, see Transplants (Facility Charges).
Transplants (Facility Charges)	Medicare covers 80% of the approved amount for transplants of the heart, lung, kidney, pancreas, intestine/multivisceral, bone marrow, cornea, and liver under certain conditions and,

---

(*continued*)

TABLE 12.1 **Medicare Coverage for the Health Care Needs of Older Adults** (*continued*)

	for some types of transplants, only at Medicare-approved facilities. Medicare only approves facilities for kidney, heart, liver, lung, intestine/multivisceral, and some pancreas transplants. Bone marrow and cornea transplants aren't limited to approved facilities. Transplant coverage includes necessary tests, labs, and exams before surgery. It also includes immunosuppressive drugs (under certain conditions), follow-up care for you, and procurement of organs and tissues. Medicare pays for the costs for a living donor for a kidney transplant.
Transportation (Routine)	Medicare generally doesn't cover transportation to get routine health care. For more information, see Ambulance Services.
Travel Outside of the United States (Health Care Coverage During Travel)	Medicare generally doesn't cover health care while you are traveling outside the United States. Puerto Rico, the U.S. Virgin Islands, Guam, American Samoa, and the Northern Mariana Islands are considered part of the United States. There are some exceptions. In some cases, Medicare may pay for services that you get while on board a ship within the territorial waters adjoining the land areas of the United States. In rare cases, Medicare can pay for inpatient hospital services that you get in a foreign country. Medicare can pay only under the following circumstances: 1. You are in the United States when a medical emergency occurs and the foreign hospital is closer than the nearest U.S. hospital that can treat the emergency. 2. You are traveling through Canada without unreasonable delay by the most direct route between Alaska and another state when a medical emergency occurs and the Canadian hospital is closer than the nearest U.S. hospital that can treat the emergency. 3. You live in the United States and the foreign hospital is closer to your home than the nearest U.S. hospital that can treat your medical condition, regardless of whether an emergency exists. Medicare also pays for doctor and ambulance services you get in a foreign country as part of a covered inpatient hospital stay.
Walker/Wheelchair	Medicare covers 80% of the cost of power-operated vehicles (scooters), walkers, and wheelchairs as DME that your doctor prescribes for use in your home. For more information, see DME. Power Wheelchair: You must have a face-to-face examination and a written prescription from a doctor or other treating provider before Medicare helps pay for a power wheelchair.
X-rays	Medicare covers medically necessary diagnostic x-rays that are ordered by your treating doctor. For more information, see Diagnostic Tests.

Source: U.S. Department of Health & Human Services Centers for Medicare & Medicaid Services (2015).

■ There are 10 standard plans that must cover some of the essentials, such as deductibles. However, each Medigap plan may also have additional benefits and set its own premiums.

■ Many traditional Medicare recipients purchase a Medigap policy. However, some older Medicare patients cannot afford the monthly premiums for these supplemental plans.

■ The Medicare Prescription Drug Improvement and Modernization Act of 2003 (also known as Medicare Part D) approved prescription discount drug cards for Medicare recipients. These cards are available to over 7 million of Medicare's 41 million participants. To be eligible for the discount cards, older adults must apply, and, depending on their income, a fee of $30 may be charged. The cards provide discounts on some, but not all, medications.

■ Culture impacts health care reimbursement in that many older adults who have immigrated to the United States live their later lives with their adult children. Those who have not paid into the U.S. Social Security system must either buy into the Medicare system (the traditional health reimbursement program for older adults) or become eligible for Medicaid. However, legislation passed in the 1990s made it more difficult for older adults who were not U.S. citizens to access Medicaid, with the result that older adults may not have any way to pay for health care.

MEDICARE MANAGED CARE, PROSPECTIVE PAYMENT SYSTEMS, AND OTHER MEDICARE SYSTEMS

■ Medicare managed care began a strong movement in the early 1990s in an attempt to lower the administrative costs associated with Medicare.

■ Medicare recipients were asked to select a health maintenance organization (HMO) from which to receive their health care.

■ Health care received through these HMOs would be paid for by Medicare.

■ Unfortunately for the HMOs, older adults used considerably more health care services than Medicare reimbursed the HMO. Consequently, HMOs lost money, and many had to withdraw from the Medicare managed care business. Although some HMOs still serve older adults in many parts of the country, many HMOs no longer take older adult Medicare clients.

■ Because of the increasing cost of health care in the 1970s and 1980s, federal legislation in 1983 implemented a prospective payment system (PPS) that involved a set payment amount before care based on the diagnosis of the patient.

■ As a result of the implementation of the PPS, older adults tend to receive more surgery and other treatments on an outpatient basis.

■ Although there are certainly positive aspects of this change in health care delivery—such as the ability to meet health care goals more effectively at home and the ability to remain free from the risks of hospitalization—should a problem arise, the need to transport to a facility with appropriate resources may be necessary, and the delay in accessing these services could increase both morbidity and mortality.

■ In further attempts to repair the problems in the Medicare system, three newer alternatives have evolved:

- Preferred provider organizations provide discounts to older adults who choose primary care providers and specialists who have agreed to accept Medicare assignment for patients.

- Medicare fee-for-service plans contract with private providers to allow older adults to go to any Medicare-approved doctor or hospital that is willing to take them. Benefits of these plans are improved coverage, such as extra hospital days. However, providers must work with private insurance plans directly to determine coverage for the health care expenditures. Moreover, an additional premium may be involved.

- Specialty plans to meet the diverse and comprehensive needs of older adults are currently being developed. More information on these plans will be available as they become more widely used among older adults.

MEDICAID

■ Medicaid, a combined federal and state payment system, varies from state to state, but it funds health care, including nursing home care, for low-income older adults.

■ Medicaid is a governmental program aimed at improving access to health care for indigent individuals.

■ Medicaid is a state-administered insurance program that provides health care for all ages. In fact, half of Medicaid recipients are children.

■ To be eligible for Medicaid, older adults must meet specific income and asset guidelines put forth by their state.

■ Older people who have minimal financial resources and who qualify for income assistance through a federal program called Supplemental Security Income (SSI) also become eligible for Medicaid health care benefits.

■ Persons age 65 and older may have Medicare benefits and also qualify for Medicaid.

■ For older adults with limited assets and income, Medicaid may supplement Medicare benefits and pay for health care expenses not covered by Medicare, including medications, additional hospital or nursing home days, and durable medical equipment.

■ For older adults who have both Medicare and Medicaid coverage for health care, Medicare is the primary payment system and Medicaid is secondary.

- The Centers for Medicare & Medicaid Services (2014) reports that Medicaid is currently the largest source of funding for health-related services for the poor in the United States.

- Medicaid was enacted by the same legislation as Medicare in 1965, also known as Title XIX of the Social Security Act.

- There is wide variability in covered medical expenses throughout the country.

- Each state establishes eligibility guidelines, allowable expenses, how much will be paid for these expenses, and how the program will be run within the state. Thus, there are as many different Medicaid programs as there are states. Mandated covered expenses for older adults include:

  - Inpatient and outpatient hospital services

  - Physician services

  - Nursing home services

  - Home care services that are delivered to prevent nursing home stays

  - Laboratory and x-ray services

- Many state Medicaid programs provide extended coverage for home- and community-based services if these services are keeping the older adult out of a covered nursing home stay; these fall within a newer Medicaid program known as All-Inclusive Care for the Elderly.

- The Personal Responsibility and Work Opportunity Reconciliation Act of a 1996 welfare reform bill made legal resident aliens and other qualified aliens who entered the United States on or after that period ineligible for Medicaid for 5 years.

- If an older adult is a Medicaid recipient, payment for health care expenses is provided directly to the health care provider.

LONG-TERM CARE INSURANCE

- Long-term care insurance is a relatively new concept designed to meet the needs of the growing elderly population.

- Approximately 7 out of 10 adults older than age 65 will need long-term care (Kaiser Family Foundation, 2013).

- More than 70% will have a length of stay of more than 3 years with an average cost of $74,000 per year. Most of the older adults cannot afford to pay out of pocket for nursing home stays.

- Consequently, an illness that results in a nursing home stay has the potential to bankrupt most middle-income older adults.

- Long-term care insurance was developed by private insurance companies to meet the long-term and chronic health care needs of older adults.

- Long-term care insurance was designed to pay for long-term health services when multiple chronic health problems occur that require custodial care not covered by Medicare or other insurance.

- There are many advantages to owning a long-term care insurance policy. But although insurance companies that offer long-term care policies are usually very ethical, they are essentially businesses with an interest in profit.

- Monthly premiums vary depending on one's age at the time of policy purchase, the length of coverage desired, the waiting period, and the desired amount of daily payments for health care expenses. Premiums are usually not fixed and may increase throughout the coverage period.

- In some cases, the premium may rise so high that older adults are no longer able to afford to pay. This may result in policy cancellation and loss of all previous monthly premiums, just when the policy benefits are needed to cover long-term nursing home, assisted living, or home care services.

- Long-term care insurance generally provides coverage for approved care in nursing facilities and assisted living.

- Care in the home by health care providers and community-based services such as care at adult day care centers are usually covered. Because the policies vary greatly, some services in these facilities may not be covered by long-term care policies.

- Long-term care insurance may be appropriate for middle-income individuals and couples who have too many financial assets to qualify for Medicaid but not enough assets to pay for long-term care.

- Because it has not been available until recently, most of the current cohort of the older adult population would be charged high premiums for coverage. Thus, long-term care insurance is rarely used to pay for long-term health care among today's older adults.

- As baby boomers begin to consider their retirement years and plan for the future, the ability to purchase long-term care insurance and use it for payment of future health care expenses will increase.

VETERANS' BENEFITS

- The Department of Veterans Affairs (VA) is a government entity that provides health care for veterans (military personnel who fought during a war).

- VA health care is provided through a network of VA medical centers, hospitals, and health facilities located across the country.

■ Once eligibility has been determined, qualified veterans may receive health care for low or no cost.

■ Eligibility for VA health care coverage, or the amount of coverage the veteran is entitled to, depends on several factors.

■ Most active-duty military personnel who served in the U.S. Army, Navy, Air Force, Marines, or Coast Guard and were honorably discharged are eligible for VA health care coverage.

■ Military reservists and National Guard members who served on active duty on order from the federal government may also be eligible for some VA health services.

■ Eligibility for health care coverage is not limited to those who served in combat. The Veterans' Health Care Eligibility Reform Act of 1996 was developed to clarify eligibility for VA health care coverage and improve health benefits for qualified beneficiaries.

■ The legislation resulted in the development of the current Uniform Benefits Package—a standard health benefits plan generally available to all veterans.

■ Once eligibility has been approved, VA health coverage under the Uniform Benefits Package is comprehensive and provides for both inpatient and outpatient coverage at VA medical centers and facilities nationwide and abroad.

■ Outpatient clinics provide physician services, primary and preventive care, diagnostic testing (including laboratory tests), minor surgery, and other needed benefits such as prescription medications.

■ The VA will also pay for hearing aids and other services after a small deductible has been met. This service is available even if the prescriptions were written by a physician other than at the VA hospital or facility.

■ Veterans with service-connected health problems are usually given priority status, but, because all veterans may receive health care at these clinics, waiting times for appointments and services may be long.

REFERENCES

Kaiser Family Foundation. (2013). A short look at long-term care for seniors. *Journal of the American Medical Association, 310*(8), 786–787. doi:10.1001/jama.2013.17676

U.S. Department of Health and Human Services, Centers for Medicare and Medicaid Services. (2015). *Medicare and you.* Bethesda, MD: Author. Retrieved March 27, 2015 from: http://www.medicare.gov/pubs/pdf/10050.pdf

13

Scope and Standards of

Geriatric Nursing Practice

LEADERSHIP AND MANAGEMENT

All gerontological nurses must be leaders in making sure they provide the highest quality care to the older adults they are responsible for, be it direct bedside care or facilitating patient care by others. Nurses need to be able to take on the following roles: creative thinker, risk taker, patient advocate, empowerer, supporter, change maker, visionary, excellent communicator, and steward (Grossman & Valiga, 2013). It is imperative that nurses be committed to making a difference, facilitating followers in gaining leadership ability, and realizing that every nurse must lead in the chaotic and challenging U.S. health care system. It is necessary to understand the differences in leadership types, such as transformational and transactional leadership. Transactional leadership tends to be evident in health care, because it involves getting the job accomplished and is very task focused. Transformational leadership involves more of an inspirational sharing between leaders and followers in which both groups are motivated and energized to perform beyond their job descriptions. Sashkin and Sashkin (2003) identify the following skills that characterize transformational leadership:

■ Ability to identify co-workers' feelings

■ Ability to motivate others

■ Ability to manage one's emotions with co-workers

By having a transformational leadership style, nurses can make a difference in their practice. Bennis (2007) suggests that exemplary leaders have six competencies that are commonly evident. They

- Create sense of mission
- Motivate followers to work with them on the mission
- Develop a social ambience for their followers
- Create trust and optimism
- Develop leadership in others
- Obtain results

Nurses working with older adults need to practice good management, which is described as being able to manage the staff and the budget, follow the organization's policies and procedures, and generate high-quality care. They are responsible for assessing, analyzing, planning, implementing, and evaluating all of the services that are part of their unit's or, in some cases, their agencies' health care delivery.

Using these skills, nurse leaders can create *culture change* within their institutions. The term *culture change* refers to a focus on high-quality individualized geriatric care that is responsive to patient needs. These institutions follow a model that frees residents from many of the issues of institutionalization (i.e., lack of autonomy and self-determination) and allows residents to engage in meaningful goal-directed activities (Burger et al., 2009).

Care that is patient or resident centered will make changes to staff schedules in order to meet individual patient care needs and preferences. Staff schedules will adjust to resident routines and may shift together with resident care needs. Resident or patient care plans and goals of care should be individualized to reflect differences in patient preferences and goals of care. Transitioning from a traditional staff-centered approach to a resident-directed approach requires organizational and managerial support.

Managers need to be effective decision makers, reflective critical thinkers, excellent time managers, and fiscal agents. Using cost–benefit analysis, nurse managers can assess the financial resources projected for costs and benefits of new programs or equipment for their unit(s). They also need to be able to foster professional development among their staff, manage conflict in all areas of their unit as well as conflict involving intra-agency unit problems. They are responsible for building teams of professional and unlicensed assistant personnel in order to have cost-efficient and cost-effective health care delivery on their unit in order to develop patient and resident-centered approaches to care.

Nurse managers need to be able to manage conflict by assisting people with their communication style (Longo, 2010). They need to encourage active listening and make sure that the team understands and shares the goal of providing the highest quality patient care. Such skills include:

- Identifying disruptive behavior
- Coaching and mentoring individuals with disruptive behavior
- Having self-awareness of how one manages conflict
- Engaging in active listening

- Creating educational incentives for nurses to identify and manage disruptive behaviors
- Fostering mutual resolution so that win–win is the overall outcome

It is essential to incorporate all of the staff when making decisions so that there will be more buy-in, and the new idea will be successful when it is implemented. The same goes for any changes that need to be made. An example of good strategizing in planning a change is explained in Sherwood's (2006) article on experiential learning, in which everyone on the unit had the opportunity to participate in making the change and having a say in what was going to happen on the unit. Due to the involvement of everyone on the staff, this change was successfully accepted.

QUALITY IMPROVEMENT

Implementing quality-improvement programs in long-term care facilities can be challenging. It is imperative that measurable outcome data are collected and tracked on clinical indicators, such as falls, medication errors, skin ulcers, infection rates, and admission/transfer rates to and from nursing homes to hospitals, so that patients can be assured that they are receiving the highest possible quality care.

The focus of many quality-of-care improvement initiatives may focus on areas where nursing care has a substantial impact on outcomes. Nursing interventions have been demonstrated to have a major impact on pressure ulcers, weight loss, reduction of the number of bedfast residents, and fall reduction.

Accreditation by The Joint Commission (previously known as both the Joint Commission on Accreditation of Healthcare Organizations or the Joint Commission on Accreditation of Hospitals) involves various audits that are assessed to validate the data that patients are experiencing high-quality care. Facilities are also assessed for performance and continued improvement in care. Audits to assess outcome, process, and structure must be done on a routine basis so that the facilities can be accredited successfully. The Centers for Medicare & Medicaid Services has similar conditions of participation that agencies caring for patients must demonstrate.

Staff nurses must be aware of the hospital quality-assurance indicators and be able to identify patients who are at high risk so more careful scrutiny can be assigned. If certain problems regarding medication or falls are occurring frequently, then interventions need to be implemented to prevent recurrences. In-services should be planned that focus on high-frequency, high-risk, and problem areas to identify the areas that staff feel they need to learn more about in order to promote high-quality and safe care in the hospital, unit, or facility. It is always prudent to conduct a needs assessment in order to determine the learning needs of staff so that they can be successful with their job duties. It is significant for nurses to be aware of the multiple assessment tools that are available to assist in the process of evaluating care and patient outcomes: the Older Americans Resources and Services Assessment measures economic resources, mental health, and activities of daily living; and the Functional Status Assessment measures a person's ability to perform his or her functions, such as activities of daily living.

There are many ideas that can be adapted from industries other than health care that can assist in improving care. For example, Six Sigma, a quality-improvement method that uses data analysis and standardized formulas to eliminate problems, has increased productivity and success at several corporations and would be easily adaptable to health care settings. Its philosophy is to prevent mistakes, waste, and redoing work.

ORGANIZATIONAL CONCEPTS

Nurses working with older adults in long-term care facilities can attend professional development classes on a variety of topics, such as the organizational structure, philosophy, goals, and objectives of the agency. Generally, the nurse manager of a unit in a long-term care facility is the director of nursing within the organizational structure and is responsible for all members of the unit staff. The facility's organizational structure illustrates the lines of communication and authority from the top administrator to the unlicensed assistive personnel and environmental assistants (Huber, 2013).

An agency's mission is the purpose and reason for its existence. The philosophy incorporates the values that guide the actions of the organization. The strategic plan identifies the long-range planning for the next 3 to 5 years. The goals and objectives of the agency describe the actions that will be taken to accomplish the strategic plan. There may be individualized unit goals that stem from the overall agency goals. The policies and procedures of an organization describe the exact processes of action that nurses should take for implementing all policies and procedures at the institution.

PROFESSIONAL DEVELOPMENT

Katz, Carter, Bishop, and Kravits (2013) describe the professional nurse as having multiple roles such as provider, health educator, advocate, case manager, change agent, manager, leader, and several similar roles at the advanced level of practice. They further define the profession as being focused on delivering holistic care to individuals, families, and communities for actual and potential health problems. All nurses have a responsibility to attend continuing-education programs and maintain their competency in practice. Many nurses have peer mentors and preceptors to assist them in maintaining their professional expertise and role models or mentors to assist them in accomplishing their career goals.

The nursing profession was the first of the health care disciplines to develop gerontological care standards for their members to demonstrate and be tested for their level of expertise. The Gerontological Nursing Board Certification exam (for which you are likely preparing) offered by the American

Nurses Credentialing Center (2014) is an example of how nursing standards of care have been developed.

Nurses can access best-practice protocols in gerontology through journals, professional organizations, gerontology conferences, and websites such as the John A. Hartford Foundation Institute for Geriatric Nursing (http://www.hartfordign.org).

LEGAL AND ETHICAL ISSUES

Regulatory Guidelines

Patients receiving care in any institution are cared for under the auspices of the Patient's Bill of Rights. Many agencies have patient ombudsmen who advocate for patients' rights. Many states have enacted right-to-die laws, and patients are able to declare their desires regarding end-of-life care in advance directives. There are statutes that control access to patient records and guarantee patient privacy, such as the Health Insurance Portability and Accountability Act.

In many instances, nurses must delegate care to others in order to accomplish the care management for older adults in long-term care and assisted living facilities. Knowing how and what can be delegated must be carefully assessed by the registered nurse. The National Council of State Boards of Nursing (NCSBN, 2005) developed the following framework of the Five Rights of Delegation that can be helpful to nurses when determining who can perform what duties:

■ Right task
■ Right circumstances
■ Right person
■ Right direction/communication
■ Right supervision

The NCSBN also delineates a process for applying the five rights of delegation when assessing a nurse's role determined by the Nurse Practice Act. Any care that a registered nurse (RN) delegates to a nursing assistant or licensed practical nurse (LPN) that is not part of the job description needs to be supervised by the RN. If the task delegated is one for which the LPN or nurse assistant has been trained, is one in which he or she can demonstrate competence, and it is in the scope of his or her practice, then the LPN or nurse assistant is accountable for his or her actions.

Many tasks can be safely and legally delegated to certified nursing assistants (CNAs). Tasks commonly delegated to CNAs include taking vital signs, applying a 12-lead EKG, measurement of I/O, collection of specimens, morning care, feeding, assisting with turning, repositioning and transfers, assistance with coughing and deep-breathing exercises, general cleaning, stocking and maintenance. Tasks that should not be delegated to CNAs include initial assessments, assessments that require specialized nursing knowledge, formulating nursing diagnoses, updating plans of care, patient education and counselling, and administering medications (American Association of Critical Care Nurses, 2004).

Ethical Principles and Decision Making

Nurses must follow ethical principles as they practice and make decisions regarding patient care. For example, every nurse should follow these principles:

■ Beneficence—Nurses should always do good and prevent harm to all patients.

■ Nonmalfeasance—Nurses must state their duty not to inflict harm.

■ Veracity—Nurses must always uphold the truth.

■ Utilitarianism—Nurses must make the decision that is positive for the most people involved.

Nurses must use the *Code of Ethics for Nurses* when they practice. This framework describes the ethical and professional values of a nurse as developed by the American Nurses Association (2001). It is important that nurses practice so that patients can be autonomous and maintain the right to make their own choices. Nurses must uphold the values that society regards as desirable (Cherry & Jacob, 2008).

Research

The research process is becoming very evident in all practice areas. Nurses are expected to be aware of the general aspects of conducting research. In fact, nurses must be able to interpret research in the literature so they can use the findings in their practice. It is important for nurses to have a general competence in understanding the quality of a research study. All nurses must understand that research is a systematic inquiry that follows disciplined methods to answer problems (Polit & Beck, 2011). Such an inquiry would include the following concepts:

■ Problem being researched—What is the background of the problem being researched?

■ Literature review—Has the author reviewed the appropriate data? Does the literature review span the findings published over the past 5 years?

■ Purpose of the research—Does the article have a specific purpose for conducting the research? Are there research questions identified that relate to the overall purpose?

■ Informed consent—Have the researchers fully informed the participants of

non-English speaking participants been communicated with in a language they understand regarding the research study? Have the authors obtained institutional review board (IRB) permission to conduct the study? Often the researchers are from universities, and they will apply for IRB consent from their university. Other times, the agency (such as a visiting nurse agency or a long-term care facility) has its own IRB from which the researchers will need to obtain approval before beginning the study.

■ Sample—Is the sample large enough? Does the sample represent the various types of people among the general population who are relevant in studying this problem? If the sample of study participants represents the general population, then the findings of the research are considered generalizable to the population.

■ Data collection—Is the study sample randomly selected or is it biased by the researchers' data-collection methods? Is it a convenience sample (i.e., were the survey participants chosen from one specific nursing home rather than a random selection of people from multiple nursing homes)?

■ Tool—Was the research tool standardized and reliable (i.e., does the tool measure what it supposed to measure), and does the tool have validity (the findings are unbiased and well grounded)? Has this tool been shown to have consistent reliability and validity?

■ Results—Are the results relevant to clinical practice? Are they going to make a difference in practice?

■ Data analysis—Are the findings statistically significant at the 0.05 level or 0.01 level? Or are they not statistically significant?

■ Discussion of findings and implications for clinical practice—Has the purpose of the study been accomplished? What else needs to be done?

Evidence-Based Practice

All nursing practice is expected to be based on emerging evidence from research, which is called evidence-based practice. Polit and Beck (2011) describe evidence-based practice as using the best possible clinical evidence to make clinical decisions for patient care. Evidence-based practice has determined that some of the "tried and true" nursing methods that have been learned from either nursing school or practice are not the best way of practicing. The best practices for gerontology can be accessed at multiple websites, such as the John A. Hartford Foundation Institute for Geriatric Nursing, http://www.hartfordign.org.

REFERENCES

American Association of Critical Care Nurses. (2004). *AACN delegation handbook* (2nd ed.). Retrieved from: http://www.aacn.org/wd/practice/docs/acndelegationhandbook.pdf

American Nurses Association. (2001). *Code of ethics for nurses with interpretive statements.*

Bennis, W. (2007). The challenges of leadership in the modern world. *American Psychologist, 62*(1), 2–5.

Burger, S. G., Kantor, B., Mezey, M., Mitty, E., Kluger, M., Algase, D., ... Rader, J. (2009). *Issue Paper: Nurses involvement in nursing home culture change: Overcoming barriers, advancing opportunities.* New York, NY: Hartford Institute for Geriatric Nursing. Retrieved October 10, 2014 from: http://hartfordign.org/uploads/File/issue_culture_change/Culture_Change_Nursing_Issue_Paper.pdf

Cherry, B., & Jacob, S. (2008). *Contemporary nursing: Issues, trends, and management* (4th ed.). St. Louis, MO: Elsevier.

Grossman, S., & Valiga, T. (2013). *The new leadership challenge: Creating the future of nursing* (4th ed.). Philadelphia, PA: F. A. Davis.

Huber, D. (2013). *Leadership and nursing care management* (5th ed.). Philadelphia, PA: Saunders.

Katz, J., Carter, C., Bishop, J., & Kravits, S. L. (2013). *Keys to nursing success* (3rd ed.). Columbus , OH: Pearson/Prentice Hall.

Longo, J., (2010). Combating disruptive behaviors: Strategies to promote a healthy work environment. *Online Journal of Issues in Nursing, 15(1),* manuscript 5.

National Council of State Boards of Nursing. (2005). *Working with others: A position paper.* Retrieved September 8, 2007, from http://www.ncsbn.org

Polit, D., & Beck, C. (2011). *Nursing research: Generating and assessing evidence for nursing practice* (9th ed.). Philadelphia, PA: Lippincott Williams & Wilkins.

Sashkin, M., & Sashkin, M. (2003). *Leadership that matters: The critical factors for making a difference in people's lives and organizations' success.* San Francisco, CA: Berrett-Koehler Publishers.

Sherwood, G. (2006). Management and leadership in nursing and health care: An experiential approach. *Journal of Continuing Education in Nursing, 37*(4), 191.

14

Posttest

1. You are performing an eye assessment of an 80-year-old man. Which of the following findings is considered abnormal?
   a. Increase in eyebrow hair due to hormonal changes
   b. The presence of arcus senilis seen around the cornea
   c. A decrease in tear production
   d. Unequal pupillary constriction in response to light

2. When discussing the increase in the number of older adults in the United States, use the term:
   a. Graying of America
   b. Maximum life span
   c. Life expectancy
   d. Total time until death

3. Tertiary prevention activities are designed to:
   a. Prevent disease before it occurs
   b. Detect disease at an earlier, more treatable stage
   c. Manage disease so it does not get worse
   d. Eradicate all disease from the nation

4. A 68-year-old woman was seen by her cardiologist for palpitations. She was put on a beta blocker and told to return for follow-up 1 week after taking a stress test. The beta blocker's action:

   a. Increases consistency of heart rate

   b. Increases contractility and decreases heart rate

   c. Decreases chance of dysrhythmia

   d. Decreases contractility and increases heart rate

5. Mary Palmer has been admitted to your unit with heart failure. Which of the following symptoms are not likely to be present in this 93-year-old woman?

   a. Cough

   b. Decreased cognitive status

   c. Fever

   d. Pedal edema

6. Herzberg is an example of what type of theory?

   a. Nursing grand theory

   b. Sociological aging theory

   c. Motivational theory

   d. Eccentricity theory

7. Mr. Gladbottle is complaining of pain, for which he needs medication. All of the following normal changes of aging should be considered when administering the medication, *except*:

   a. Increased excretion through the urinary tract

   b. Decreased absorption from the gastrointestinal tract

   c. Decreased metabolism of medications

   d. Decreased renal clearance

8. You have just admitted an 88-year-old man to the long-term care facility. He is on several medications, including allopurinol (Zyloprim) and bethanechol (Urecholine), which are for:

   a. Arthritis

   b. Amyotrophic lateral sclerosis

   c. Gout

   d. Polyarteritis

9. A new staff nurse is orienting to the long-term care facility. The staff development coordinator will be sure to include time for the new nurse to review the institution's:

   a. Plan for developing new funding for the facility

   b. Listing of each staff member's salary

   c. Mission, philosophy, and goals of the organization

   d. The next 6 months' scheduling of nursing assistants on each unit

10. A 68-year-old resident of an assisted living facility complains of muscle aches and loss of range of motion in multiple joints, especially in his left knee. He says he is sexually active and has multiple partners. His temperature is 99.1°C; he has no tophi on his left knee, but it is warm and swollen. The etiology of his knee pain is:

    a. Severe osteopenia or osteoporosis

    b. Septic arthritis secondary to gonorrhea and chlamydia

    c. Sarcoidosis

    d. Osteomyelitis

11. The *absence* of which of the following symptoms makes diagnosis of pneumonia difficult in older adults?

    a. Bradycardia

    b. Tachycardia

    c. Cough

    d. Cyanosis

12. The nurse manager of a geriatric unit has been having trouble motivating the staff on her unit and recently received low patient and nurse satisfaction scores. The other RNs on this unit are transferring to other units whenever there are open positions. This manager is noted for her authoritarian leadership and strong task-oriented style. She reflects which of the following types of leadership?

    a. Democratic

    b. Transformational

    c. Transactional

    d. Laissez-faire

13. It may take several weeks for the postherpetic pain secondary to herpes zoster experienced by many older adults to subside. Therefore, it is recommended that a pain medication and which of the following therapies be used?

    a. Magnet therapy

    b. Continued acyclovir (Zovirax)

    c. Meperidine (Demerol)

    d. Capsaicin cream

14. A 77-year-old man presents to the emergency department in acute pain. He says he has new-onset left leg pain and that his leg is really swollen with erythematous streaks. He is diagnosed with:

    a. Gout

    b. Rheumatoid arthritis

    c. Cellulitis

    d. Fibromyalgia

15. If a study is said to use a random sampling, this means the sample was:

    a. Representative of the average American

    b. Chosen on the basis of convenience

    c. Determined using clustering technique to ensure homogeneity

    d. Selected so that each member of a population has an equal probability of being included

16. The degree to which a patient follows a treatment regimen could best be defined as:

    a. Adherence

    b. Health literacy

    c. Deliverance

    d. Holism

17. Due to the fact that there can be under- and overestimates of an individual's abilities, it is best to use which of the following as the primary source of information in an older adult assessment?

    a. Primary care provider

    b. The spouse or child of the older adult

    c. The older adult

    d. The executor of the older adult's estate

18. Restraints should rarely be used in long-term care facilities. However, which of the following situations is an acceptable reason for using restraints on an older adult?

    a. When the patient wants to get out of bed and go to the bathroom several times a night

    b. When the patient is restless and has no order for a sedative

    c. When the patient becomes agitated after meals

    d. To ensure the physical safety of the patient or other patients

19. Posttransplant, the chance for developing acute graft-versus-host disease tends to fall:

    a. During the first 20 days posttransplant

    b. Within the first 24 hours posttransplant

    c. Between 3 and 6 months posttransplant

    d. Within the first week posttransplant

20. Which of the following points would the nurse include in teaching an older adult who is beginning an exercise program?

    a. Begin an exercise program with 30 to 60 minutes of vigorous exercise each day

    b. Avoid drinking water when exercising

    c. Keep a daily written log of exercise and include type of exercise, time of exercise, and the intensity of exercise

    d. Dizziness is common when exercising and should be ignored

21. To obtain a patient's informed consent to participate in a research study, prior to enrolling patients in a research project, the researcher must obtain approval from:

    a. Nurses working with the patient

    b. Patient's family members

    c. Long-term care facility attorney

    d. Institutional review board

22. An 88-year-old man complains of burning on the soles of his feet. He has a complete physical examination and has no other significant findings. His laboratory work returns with a decrease in:

    a. Vitamin C

    b. Vitamin B$_{12}$

    c. Iron

    d. Potassium

23. Mrs. Crotwell is a 90-year-old woman who has been hospitalized with a medical diagnosis of osteoporosis. Which of the following is most likely her primary form of insurance?

    a. COBRA

    b. Medicare

    c. Medicaid

    d. HUSKY

24. The end of life is often associated with which of the following psychological symptoms among older adults?

    a. Anxiety

    b. Cough

    c. Shortness of breath

    d. Pain

25. An 81-year-old man has been experiencing some memory loss over the past year, but today he got lost driving to his son's home. He has had various laboratory tests, neuroimaging, and cognitive testing and has been diagnosed with Alzheimer's disease. Due to his increasing dementia, he is being discharged to his son's home. The priority intervention that must be promoted is:

    a. Protection from injury

    b. Behavior modification

    c. Independence with activities of daily living

    d. Memory restoration

26. The purpose of the Health Insurance Portability and Accountability Act (HIPAA) is to:

    a. Provide reimbursement for prescriptions

    b. Set up insurance policies for emergencies

    c. Provide older adults guaranteed access to health care

    d. Protect patient privacy

27. In the continuity theory of aging:

    a. Successful aging is an extension of an individual's developmental patterns throughout life

    b. Aging should be denied as long as possible

    c. Cells divide continually a predetermined number of times, and then death occurs

    d. Products of oxidation result in a breakdown of cells, and the body slowly begins to age

28. Many older adults have osteoarthritis resulting in painful hips and knees. An appropriate intervention for them is:

   a. Application of heat and/or cold, whichever is effective

   b. NSAIDs with food every 2 hours

   c. Steroids twice daily

   d. Cortisone injections twice daily

29. Older adults with pneumonia are three to five times more likely than younger patients with pneumonia to experience which of the following?

   a. Cardiovascular collapse

   b. Complications leading to death

   c. Fever less than 105°F

   d. Acute renal failure

30. A characteristic of delirium is:

   a. Intellectual dysfunction that occurs slowly and lasts for longer than 6 months

   b. Decreased severity at nighttime disorientation

   c. A progressive decline in memory

   d. Disorientation

31. A 66-year-old presents with a purple-colored papular rash on his face. He is HIV positive and states that the rash is worsening, he has never experienced it before, and, although painless, it is causing concern. The rash is:

   a. Psoriasis

   b. Tinea capitis

   c. Impetigo

   d. Kaposi's sarcoma

32. A 77-year-old man has recently been diagnosed with early heart failure. He will most likely be prescribed which of the following?

   a. Digoxin

   b. ACE inhibitor

   c. Calcium channel blocker

   d. Beta blocker

33. A 75-year-old man is sightseeing in Arizona and finds that he is extremely thirsty in the hot climate. This is due to less ability to conserve fluid and concentrate urine. Therefore, one would expect:

    a. Increased glomerular filtration rate (GFR)

    b. Decreased blood urea nitrogen (BUN) and creatinine

    c. Decreased GFR

    d. Increased erythropoietin

34. Primary prevention activities are designed to:

    a. Prevent disease before it occurs

    b. Detect disease at an earlier, more treatable stage

    c. Manage disease so it does not get worse

    d. Eradicate all disease from the nation

35. Common musculoskeletal problems for older adults include which of the following?

    a. Paget's disease and osteomyelitis

    b. Bunions and corns on feet

    c. Osteoarthritis and osteoporosis

    d. Rheumatoid arthritis and plantar fasciitis

36. Older adults often don't report pain because:

    a. They believe that pain is a normal part of aging

    b. They are afraid of what the pain might mean

    c. They don't want to bother the nurse

    d. All of the above

37. Older adults tend to have increased dental problems due to:

    a. Periodontal disease

    b. Changes in pH of saliva

    c. Decreased fluid needs

    d. Less mucus excreted from salivary glands

38. Ways in which geriatric nurses may help older patients fulfill their spiritual needs at the end of life may include:

    a. Ignore spiritual needs because these are best managed by other team members

    b. Focus on pain management

    c. Focus on maintaining adequate oxygenation

    d. Encourage religious and spiritual practices at the end of life

39. Practice that focuses on making decisions clinically using the best evidence available is called:

a. Applied research practice

b. Research utilization practice

c. Evidence-based practice

d. Empirical evidence practice

40. A 66-year-old man has recently been diagnosed with Ménière's disease and is experiencing another episode. His symptoms will include:

a. Decreased hearing and difficulty with balance

b. Pain in the outer ear and itchiness

c. Shrill sounds upon talking and decreased hearing

d. Dizziness and tinnitus

41. Older adults suffering from early dementia due to Alzheimer's disease are generally prescribed a cholinesterase inhibitor. The action of these drugs is to:

a. Decrease catecholamine surges

b. Increase the brain's level of acetylcholine

c. Decrease serotonin uptake

d. Increase norepinephrine levels

42. The organizational structure of any facility represents the:

a. Line of authority from the administrator to the unlicensed assistive personnel

b. Line of authority for the nursing personnel only

c. Process by which the organization is departmentalized

d. Categories of employees

43. Title III of the Older Americans Act facilitated the start of:

a. Centers for Medicare & Medicaid Services

b. AARP

c. Area Agencies on Aging

d. Gerontological Society of America

44. Forty percent to sixty percent of older adults have anemia due to iron deficiency or some chronic illness. Additionally, many medications can cause anemia. Which of the following drug categories can cause gastrointestinal bleeding if not taken with food?

    a. Anticonvulsants

    b. Antihypertensives

    c. NSAIDs

    d. Diuretics

45. The febrile response of older adults to infection:

    a. Is about the same as that of a young child

    b. Is blunted with age

    c. Is always greater than that of younger adults

    d. Depends on the type of thermometer used

46. A 73-year-old woman has osteoarthritis in multiple joints. She has an especially difficult time with fine motor work and has recently been diagnosed with:

    a. Veritas erythema

    b. Bouchard's nodules

    c. Heberden's nodes

    d. Hallux valgus

47. One of the most influential advocacy groups for older adults is:

    a. Centers for Medicare & Medicaid Services

    b. AARP

    c. Association on Aging

    d. Gerontological Society of America

48. A nursing intervention in a geriatric care plan:

    a. Describes nursing actions that will assist the patient to meet the identified goals

    b. Must be broad enough so that any member of the health care team can modify them if necessary

    c. Is based on the medical diagnosis

    d. Organizes the data obtained in the assessment

49. The guideline used to determine the relative safety of medications for older adults is:

  a. Cogs Criteria

  b. Glasgow Scale

  c. Beers Criteria

  d. Ramsey's Scale

50. Many variables cause the increased risk of incontinence in older adults. Which of the following is a normal change of aging that impacts one's urinary continence?

  a. Decreased ability to mobilize

  b. Decreased cognition

  c. Decreased bladder capacity

  d. Depression

51. Which of these statements, if made by the older adult, would be most likely to be an indicator of depression?

  a. "I feel like I have accomplished something today"

  b. "I am just too tired to do anything"

  c. "I would like to visit my daughter"

  d. "My life has had many ups and downs"

52. An 83-year-old man presents with hyperlipidemia with the following laboratory results: TC 242, high-density lipoprotein (HDL) 54, low-density lipoprotein (LDL) 168, and TG 110. He has well-controlled hypertension and no other history. Which of the parameters should be focused on for management?

  a. HDL should be higher

  b. LDL should be less than 100

  c. Triglycerides should be lower

  d. Total cholesterol should be around 240

53. Which of the following would be an appropriate activity for the RN to delegate to the unlicensed assistive personnel?

  a. Medication administration

  b. Nutritional assessment

  c. Bathing

  d. Admission documentation

54. Secondary prevention activities are designed to:
    a. Prevent disease before it occurs
    b. Detect disease at an earlier, more treatable stage
    c. Manage disease so it does not get worse
    d. Eradicate all disease from the nation

55. A set of national health objectives designed to guide the health promotion activities of the United States is known as:
    a. Healthy People 1998
    b. Healthy People 2020
    c. A Sick Nation
    d. Blueprint for Health

56. Stress incontinence is common among older adults who can benefit from doing which of these specific exercises?
    a. Bicellular stretches
    b. Detrusor splints
    c. Kegel exercises
    d. Perineum exercises

57. Durable power of attorney provides which information if a patient should experience a terminal condition or a permanent state of unconsciousness?
    a. Written information describing the patient's desires for life-sustaining treatment
    b. Names a person for making health care decisions on behalf of the patient
    c. Provides information for the distribution of the patient's financial assets
    d. Provides for terminal care at the end of life

58. Older adults tend to have increased blood pressures because of their:
    a. Decreased oral intake
    b. Increased cardiac output
    c. Increased blood flow
    d. Decreased vascular compliance

59. An 81-year-old man has been experiencing temporal headaches and has been seen by his physician and diagnosed with temporal arteritis. He has most likely been prescribed:

    a. Azithromycin (Z-pak)

    b. Ibuprofen (Advil)

    c. Prednisone

    d. Sumatriptan (Imitrex)

60. A 67-year-old man presents with red blotches, papules, and pustules on his face, especially over his chin and cheek areas. He says he does not remember ever having this problem before. This is most likely:

    a. Folliculitis

    b. Acne vulgaris

    c. Eczema

    d. Rosacea

61. A 76-year-old woman has postop craniotomy due to a benign tumor. She is febrile, has odorous drainage, and her incision is erythematous and indurated. You suspect she is infected and find that your older patients often experience infection postoperatively. This is due to:

    a. Fewer killer T cells in the immunologic system

    b. Inflammation due to increased cytokines

    c. Weaker neutrophil response to infection

    d. Cortisol deficiency

62. Health care costs for older adults have increased greatly as a result of which of the following factors?

    a. Increased cost of medication

    b. Decreased educational levels of the elderly

    c. Decreased numbers of older adults

    d. The nursing shortage

63. It is most important to teach older adults with type 2 diabetes about the relationship of postprandial glucose levels and:

    a. Carbohydrates

    b. Fats

    c. Proteins

    d. Iron

64. In discussing the biological theories of aging, the nurse would include information on which of the following theories?

   a. The "wear and tear" theory

   b. The disengagement theory

   c. The continuity theory

   d. The activity theory

65. It is not uncommon for older adults who experience influenza to have persistent problems afterward, such as:

   a. Anemia, chest discomfort, and cough

   b. Lack of energy, fatigue, and malaise

   c. Fatigue, anemia, and myalgia

   d. Malaise, fever, and cough

66. It is essential to realize that older adults must get an adequate dietary intake of which the following elements due to the fact that aging causes a decrease in absorption of this element in the gastrointestinal system?

   a. Potassium

   b. Sodium

   c. Hydrogen

   d. Iron

67. Mr. and Mrs. Suhul live in an assisted living facility and rarely leave their apartment. They have recently said that they feel depressed and lethargic and ask you about the facility's social activities. You suggest that they:

   a. Make appointments with the psychiatrist

   b. Sign up for an exercise class, get some sun, and do yoga

   c. Add more protein to their diets

   d. Get a vitamin C supplement

68. An older patient is preparing for discharge on warfarin (Coumadin) 5 mg orally every day. He asks you if he should continue with his multivitamin when he gets home. Your response is:

   a. "It is fine to take a multivitamin daily"

   b. "If there is no vitamin K in it, you can take it"

   c. "You should take two multivitamins daily"

   d. "It is best to take the multivitamin before you go to sleep"

69. In assessing pain in older adults, nurses must realize that:

   a. Older adults are quicker to report pain than younger adults

   b. Pain is a normal consequence of aging

   c. An elderly person may not exhibit outward signs of pain even when he or she is actually experiencing pain

   d. Pain is rated on a scale of 0 to 10, with 10 being no feelings of pain and 0 being the most severe pain

70. Older adults are frequently diagnosed with anemia of chronic disease, which is commonly seen with which of the following?

   a. Cardiovascular and pulmonary disease

   b. Renal and neurological problems

   c. Malignancies and tuberculosis

   d. Musculoskeletal and neurological problems

71. Nurses must complete a core set of screening and assessment elements that form the foundation of the comprehensive assessment used for their home care residents. This assessment tool is called the:

   a. Minimum Data Set (MDS)

   b. OASIS assessment

   c. Resident assessment set

   d. Maximum dependency scale

72. Some older adults withhold medical information or details about their living arrangements, because they:

   a. May feel the care provider is not really interested in all of the details

   b. May not realize that some of this information would be helpful for planning their care

   c. May not remember all of the details of their medical history or living arrangements

   d. All of the above

73. Some older adults manifest changes in their skin that appear as light brown macules on the dorsum of their hand, wrist, and forearm called:

   a. Actinic keratosis

   b. Skin tags

   c. Rosacea

   d. Seborrheic dermatitis

74. Mr. H., an 81-year-old man, has an HDL of 75. Your teaching for him would include instructions to:

    a. Decrease his intake of eggs and whole-milk products

    b. Decrease the amount of glucose in his diet

    c. Take cholinesterase as prescribed

    d. Keep up the good work!

75. Quality-improvement indicators for facilities for older adults need to monitor which of the following types of high-risk and problem-prone areas?

    a. Fall risk and body image

    b. Adverse effects of polypharmacy

    c. Fall risk, body image, and hydration status

    d. Hydration status, hip injuries, and hearing needs

76. The aging process increases the chance of older adults experiencing presbyopia that causes difficulty focusing on near objects. This is due to:

    a. Inflammation of the cornea

    b. Trauma to the vitreous humor

    c. Pupil reaction time

    d. Loss of elasticity of the lens

77. Many older adults take NSAIDs for discomfort. It is extremely important to monitor which of the following systems for serious side effects?

    a. Integumentary

    b. Neurological

    c. Reproductive

    d. Gastrointestinal

78. Some older adults have a higher frequency of developing GERD due to:

    a. Increased esophageal muscle spasticity

    b. Effects of multiple medications they take

    c. Incompetent lower esophageal sphincter

    d. Decrease in HCL secretion

79. If verbal statements provide information for advance directives and are provided by the patient to the geriatric nurse, the best way to make sure they are followed is to:

    a. Tell them to as many people as possible

    b. Check them with the family

c. Document them

d. Don't do anything because they may conflict with families' desires for patients at the end of life

80. Due to aging changes in the immunologic system such as decreased cell functioning ability, older adults are at risk for which of the following?

   a. Infection

   b. Immunological mutation

   c. Thrombocytopenia

   d. Anemia

81. The percentage of older adults in nursing homes who are in pain has been reported to be as high as:

   a. 10%

   b. 30%

   c. 50%

   d. 85%

82. The purpose of obtaining certification as a gerontological nurse is to:

   a. Establish a minimal level of professional competency

   b. Recognize excellence in practice

   c. Demonstrate advanced nursing practice level of competency

   d. Identify one's readiness for RN licensure

83. Mrs. Pipekettle, a 79-year-old woman, had a hysterectomy last night. She was transferred to your unit from recovery this morning and has been yelling and trying to remove her bandages all day long. The reason for this is most likely:

   a. Dementia

   b. Delirium

   c. Depression

   d. Bipolar disease

84. Frequent dermatological lesions experienced by the elderly include:

   a. Cherry angiomas, senile lentigines (liver spots), and skin tags

   b. Lichen planus, acne, and pityriasis rosea

   c. Warts, moles, and acne

   d. Melanoma, warts, and cherry angiomas

85. Living wills provide which information if a patient should experience a terminal condition or a permanent state of unconsciousness?

    a. Written information describing the patient's desires for life-sustaining treatment

    b. Names a person for making health care decisions on behalf of the patient

    c. Information for the distribution of the patient's financial assets

    d. Provisions for terminal care at the end of life

86. It is difficult to perform a pelvic exam on some older women because of:

    a. Vaginal atrophy and dryness

    b. Introitus shrinkage

    c. Labia minora and majora stretching

    d. Vaginal canal elongation

87. An example of primary prevention is:

    a. Breast cancer screening

    b. Diabetes disease management

    c. Annual prostate-specific antigen (PSA) testing

    d. Smoking cessation

88. Risk factors for osteoporosis include all of the following, *except*:

    a. Active lifestyle

    b. Family history

    c. Early menopause

    d. Caucasian or Asian ancestry

89. Older adults with diabetes mellitus experience macrovascular and microvascular complications. Some of the microvascular complications include:

    a. Hypertension, stroke, and myocardial infarction

    b. Peripheral vascular disease, venous stasis, and amputation

    c. Renal dysfunction, neuropathy, and retinopathy

    d. Stroke, pulmonary embolism, and amputation

90. A 78-year-old nursing home resident is prescribed isoniazid for a positive purified protein test (+PPD). He is also given a prescription for vitamin B_6 to prevent:

    a. Uveitis

    b. Peripheral neuropathy

    c. Meningitis

    d. Trigeminal neuralgia

91. The purpose of ethnogeriatrics is:

    a. Ignoring cultural practices because all people have basically the same needs

    b. Developing cultural competence in the care of older adults

    c. Spending minimal time in the patient's room when there is a language barrier so as not to confuse the patient

    d. Avoiding the use of an interpreter in order to help the patient learn a different language

92. New-onset seizures can occur with young or older adults. With older adults the most frequent cause of seizures is:

    a. Cerebrovascular disease

    b. Pulmonary disease

    c. Immunological deficiency

    d. Electrolyte imbalance

93. The nurse discusses a core set of screening and assessment elements that form the foundation of the comprehensive assessment for all residents of long-term care facilities. This assessment tool is called the:

    a. MDS

    b. OASIS

    c. Resident Assessment Set

    d. Maximum Dependency Scale

94. Geriatric facilities should conduct quality-improvement measurements on which of the following outcomes?

    a. Medication errors, falls, skin breakdown, and infection rates

    b. Rate of polypharmacy, incident report rate, and nurse satisfaction

    c. Number of medications used per patient, infection rate, and falls

    d. Falls, patient gender, and nurse education

95. Due to the increase in anterior–posterior diameter of the thorax from the aging process, one will typically elicit which of the following sounds with percussion when assessing older adults?

    a. Flat

    b. Dull

    c. Resonance

    d. Hyperresonance

96. First-line disease-modifying drugs for rheumatoid arthritis include:

    a. Tylenol, Aleve

    b. Percocet, phenobarbitol

    c. Methotrexate, hydroxychloroquine (Plaquenil)

    d. Elavil, Prozac

97. Four members of an assisted living facility's chess team complain of seeing colored rings around the lights and have been having a difficult time seeing the chess pieces and the board. These individuals need to see an ophthalmologist for:

    a. Astigmatism

    b. Macular degeneration

    c. Glaucoma

    d. Retinal detachment

98. Harriet Gray has developed a decubitus ulcer on her coccyx. All of the following risk factors may have caused this, *except:*

    a. Orthopnea

    b. Moisture

    c. Inactivity

    d. Shearing

99. When performing a functional assessment on an 82-year-old client with a recent stroke, which of the following questions would be most important to ask?

    a. "Do you wear glasses?"

    b. "Do you have any thyroid medication?"

    c. "How many times a day do you have a bowel movement?"

    d. "Are you able to dress yourself?"

100. The most commonly seen leukemia in older adults is:
   a. Acute lymphocytic leukemia
   b. Chronic lymphocytic leukemia
   c. Acute myelogenic leukemia
   d. Chronic lymphocytic leukemia

101. A research tool that has strong reliability indicates that it is able to:
   a. Measure an attribute consistently
   b. Correlate the dependent variables with each other
   c. Assess the participant's knowledge about a topic
   d. Monitor how the environment is impacting the participants' responses

102. Which of the following are valid tools for assessing pain?
   a. SF-36 Short Form
   b. Faces Pain Scale
   c. Geriatric Depression Scale (GDS)
   d. Mini-Mental Exam

103. Older adults are prone to which of the following side effects of opiates, tricyclic antidepressants, and anticholinergics?
   a. Diarrhea
   b. Abdominal cramping
   c. Muscular aches
   d. Constipation

104. Which of the following age-related changes may affect older adults' ability to respond to cold temperatures?
   a. Increased cardiac output
   b. Increased subcutaneous tissue
   c. Decreased peripheral circulation
   d. Increased muscle mass

105. An example of an outcomes audit would be:

    a. Testing the nurses regarding their knowledge of high-risk indicators

    b. Measuring the number of patients who had falls in their bedrooms

    c. Surveying the patients for their perceptions of how well the nurse administrator does his or her job

    d. Providing outcome data to the families regarding health care

106. Laurie Gunther is considered a pioneer of aging research for her work in the field of gerontological nursing during the:

    a. 1940s

    b. 1950s

    c. 1960s

    d. 1970s

107. Body mass index (BMI) is determined by calculating one's weight and height and using a BMI calculator wheel by plugging in the weight and height to determine BMI. A normal BMI for an older adult would be:

    a. 30 or higher

    b. 25 to 29.9

    c. 18.5 to 24.9

    d. Below 18.5

108. Infection is more difficult to assess in older adults because they tend not to be able to manifest the typical symptoms of infection, including which of the following?

    a. Fever and increased white blood cell count

    b. Increased red blood cells and increased platelets

    c. Fever and increased platelets

    d. Heat rash and tachypnea

109. Older adults have a decreased ability to respond to dim light due to decreased retinal illumination with aging. A good example of this is when an older adult goes into a dark movie theater after the movie has started. The person should be sure to:

    a. Take extra time to adapt to the dim light before trying to find a seat

    b. Get new prescriptive lenses to assist with the adaptation to darkness

    c. Never go alone into a dark setting

    d. Avoid darkened settings entirely

110. Spiritual care begins with:

   a. A plan of care

   b. Assessment

   c. Diagnosis of spiritual distress

   d. Discharge planning

111. The primary source of payment for older adult health care is:

   a. Medicare

   b. Medicaid

   c. Private insurance

   d. Medigap

112. Due to the physiological changes in the pulmonary system, such as decreased vital capacity, decreased gas exchange, and decreased cough reflex, older postoperative patients are more likely to experience:

   a. Pulmonary embolus and pleuritis

   b. Pneumonia and atelectasis

   c. Pleural effusion and pneumothorax

   d. Bronchiectasis and rib fracture

113. Nurses must be aware of which of the following age-related changes that affect continence?

   a. An increase in the bladder capacity

   b. A decrease in bladder muscle tone, which results in a lessened ability to postpone voiding

   c. A decrease in residual volume to less than 20 mL

   d. An increased perception of the sensation of the urge to void

114. A 78-year-old man presents to the emergency department with a complaint of dizziness whenever he stands up. He has been diagnosed with benign prostate hyperplasia and has been taking doxazosin (Cardura) for approximately 2 weeks. Your priority action is to:

   a. Discuss time of administration with the patient

   b. Perform orthostatic blood pressure and pulse assessment

   c. Prepare him for intravenous hydration

   d. Teach him the benefits of a low-sodium diet

115. Approximately what percentage of hospice patients are considered older adults?

    a. 25%

    b. 50%

    c. 75%

    d. 100%

116. An example of a standard tool of assessment used frequently with older adults to plan high-quality care is:

    a. Medicaid survey

    b. Medicare assessment

    c. Older American Resources and Services Assessment

    d. Geriatric Activity Tool

117. Older adults who are bed- or chair-bound experience decubitus ulcers on their bony prominences more so than younger patients. The general sequence of manifestations is:

    a. Maceration of skin, edema, ulceration

    b. Macular rash, blistering, ulceration

    c. Ecchymosis, erythema, ulceration

    d. Erythema, edema, ulceration

118. An 88-year-old woman complains of shoulder pain that has been increasing over the past 6 months. She is assessed and diagnosed with impingement syndrome, which is most likely a result of:

    a. Frozen shoulder

    b. Wearing an arm sling for longer than 3 months

    c. Rotator cuff tendonitis

    d. Thoracic outlet syndrome

119. Which of the following is a classical ethical principle often employed in gerontology?

    a. Malpractice

    b. Competency

    c. Beneficence

    d. Accountability

120. The most common type of hearing loss among older adults is:

   a. Presbycusis

   b. Lipidocusis

   c. Ménière's disease

   d. Arcus senilus

121. It is not uncommon for older adults to experience fecal incontinence caused by changes in the gastrointestinal system such as:

   a. Increased peristalsis

   b. Loss of sphincter control

   c. Increased tonicity of anal column

   d. Diverticulosis

122. A 65-year-old man has a history of using Percocet and nonsteroidal anti-inflammatory drugs (NSAIDs) for lower back pain. He drinks three beers daily and more on weekends. He notes that he is turning yellow, feels confused, is dizzy, and has no energy. When he notices that he has bright red blood in the toilet after a bowel movement, he presents to the emergency department. Your priority concern is:

   a. Referral to the transplant coordinator

   b. To stabilize his vital signs and give fluid resuscitation

   c. To assess his mental status to establish a baseline

   d. Pain management

123. One of the greatest barriers to successful interventions to help older problem drinkers is that:

   a. Older adults don't usually drive, so intoxication while driving is not detected.

   b. Nurses and health care professionals fail to detect problem alcohol use.

   c. Many of the medications taken by older adults mimic the effects of alcohol.

   d. Alcoholism occurs so rarely in the elderly that interventions are usually not necessary.

124. The use of histamine H_2 blockers can cause problems with older adults because of drug interactions with the numerous medications they take and other central nervous system side effects. An example of these H_2 receptor blockers is:

    a. Cimetidine (Tagamet)

    b. Clarithromycin (Biaxin)

    c. Raloxifene (Evista)

    d. Fexofenadine (Allegra)

125. Medicare and Medicaid legislation is important for all of the following reasons *except:*

    a. It provides health care coverage for the most vulnerable segments of U.S. society

    b. It was an initial step toward federal health care coverage.

    c. It built on the Social Security Act.

    d. It was the first federal health care legislation to be broadly supported by the American Medical Association.

126. The increase in the older adult population will likely:

    a. Stabilize in the future

    b. Continue for some years to come

    c. Stop by the year 2030

    d. Be impossible to predict

127. A 77-year-old woman has been admitted for heart failure. You prepare her for a blood draw that includes a complete blood count with differential and which of the following?

    a. CA-125 and C-reactive protein

    b. Brain natriuretic peptide and complete chemistry profile

    c. ANA titer and electrolytes

    d. CA-33 and complete chemistry profile

128. A 76-year-old diabetic woman has a hemoglobin A1c of 8.9, so she is going to be started on glargine (Lantus) insulin. What would the administration be?

    a. With meals

    b. Once a day

    c. Before breakfast and dinner

    d. At bedtime

129. Men experience andropause with the gradual decline in testosterone and other hormones as they age. Erectile dysfunction is not a normal part of the aging process but rather is due to what condition?

    a. Immunological dysfunction

    b. Cardiovascular dysfunction

    c. Renal dysfunction

    d. Dermatologic dysfunction

130. Older adults have a high frequency of folic acid deficiency anemia, which is often the result of:

    a. Poor nutrition

    b. Genetic factors

    c. Coagulopathy

    d. Inflammation

131. A family caregiver has been caring for her elderly mother for several years. The caregiver is becoming very tired from the 24-hour-a-day responsibility of caring for her mother. The nurse would most likely suggest which of the following alternatives first?

    a. Acute care

    b. Hospice care

    c. Placing her mother in a nursing home

    d. Respite care

132. Regarding sexuality in older adults, nurses should know that:

    a. Sexuality is not an important part of older adults' lives

    b. Impotence is a natural occurrence with age

    c. A number of chronic illnesses affect the sexual function of the elderly

    d. Men older than 75 years of age are incapable of fathering a child

133. Health care institutions in some states must provide advance directives to their patients. This means that:

    a. The institution believes in euthanasia.

    b. The patients can declare their desires regarding end-of-life care.

    c. The patients will receive a full resuscitation if the situation requires it.

    d. No do-not-resuscitate decisions can be made.

134. Older adults with asthma frequently have viral infections prior to experiencing which of the following?

    a. Acute emphysema

    b. Pneumonia

    c. Acute exacerbations of their asthma

    d. Acute respiratory failure

135. A 70-year-old woman is being discharged to her home after being hospitalized for management of her bradycardia. She tells you that she has recently gained weight, lost all of her energy, always feels tired, and experiences general muscle aches and pains in her extremities. She tells you that the cardiologist is having her see her primary care provider for a workup because he found some abnormal laboratory results regarding her thyroid. You are not surprised that she is diagnosed with:

    a. Hyperthyroidism

    b. Multinodular goiter

    c. Hypothyroidism

    d. Graves' disease

136. Ms. Lee, age 65, is worried about developing osteoporosis. Which of the following assessment findings would indicate that she may be at risk for osteoporosis?

    a. She exercises at least three times per week.

    b. She drinks three to four glasses of milk per day.

    c. She is Asian.

    d. She enjoys an occasional glass of wine.

137. An 87-year-old man asks you to explain what the action of losartan (Cozaar) is. Your explanation is that the drug:

    a. Prevents high blood pressure

    b. Promotes the excretion of potassium

    c. Blocks the actions of angiotensin II

    d. Prevents the secretion of natriuretic peptide

138. It is imperative that health care providers ask older adults about which common problems of aging?

    a. Financial resources, ability to communicate with neighbors, and musculoskeletal disorders

    b. Depression, dementia, urinary function, and health literacy

c. Financial resources, urinary function, and history of drug abuse

d. Anxiety, depression, bipolar disorder, and schizophrenia

139. Normal changes of aging that affect older adults include which of the following?

a. Loss of teeth

b. Changes in senses of smell and taste

c. Loneliness and social isolation

d. All of the above

140. Mr. Foley, age 88, has lived with his son, daughter-in-law, and grandchildren for 5 years. He has recently been very afraid of the dark, the neighbors, and his grandchildren. He is afraid someone is trying to hurt him. This condition is most likely described as:

a. Depression

b. Paranoia

c. Amnesia

d. Memory loss

141. When older adults cannot afford health care, they often become _____ with treatment plans of care.

a. Angry

b. Noncompliant

c. Disgruntled

d. Frustrated

142. Religion is defined as:

a. A framework within which older adults search for meaning and purpose in life

b. An organized system of beliefs, practices, and rituals designed to foster closeness to a sacred reality

c. A means by which older adults complete developmental tasks of aging

d. A means by which older adults accomplish physical dimensions of aging

143. The nurses at a long-term care facility are having difficulty implementing a new wound procedure. Many of the nurses are unfamiliar with the procedure and are notifying you that they do not feel comfortable performing the wound care. What would you do if you were the director of nursing?

    a. Ask the nurses to collaborate with each other regarding the new procedure.

    b. Have the medical director teach the nurses about the wound care.

    c. Have one nurse volunteer to develop and teach the wound care after learning it from a wound care consultant who is familiar with the procedure.

    d. Call another long-term care facility and ask how to perform the wound care.

144. When a medical diagnosis cannot be found for chronic malnutrition among older adults, nurses may consider the possibility of which syndrome?

    a. Polypharmacy

    b. Hypertension

    c. Failure to thrive

    d. Gall stones

145. It is not uncommon for older adults to experience systolic which kind of murmurs?

    a. Aortic stenosis

    b. Aortic regurgitation

    c. Mitral stenosis

    d. Systolic pan murmur

146. An 86-year-old man has scaly, horny lesions on his trunk. This is most likely:

    a. Contact dermatitis

    b. Seborrheic keratosis

    c. Actinic keratosis

    d. Lichen planus

147. A research tool that has strong reliability indicates that it is able to:

    a. Measure an attribute consistently.

    b. Correlate the dependent variables with each other.

c. Assess the participant's knowledge about a topic.

d. Monitor how the environment is impacting the participant's responses.

148. Cardiovascular changes coincident with aging affect the endothelial walls of the vessels because of:

a. Increased levels of collagen

b. Increased elasticity

c. Decreased levels of elastin

d. Decreased levels of calcium

149. A 66-year-old patient newly diagnosed with type 2 diabetes mellitus asks why she has to take insulin when her friends take oral drugs for their diabetes. Her fasting blood sugar was 220 and she had been experiencing polydipsia, polyphagia, and polyuria. Your answer includes which of the following explanations?

a. Insulin will provide the quickest way to reach the optimum glycemic target for you.

b. The oral agents are far too dangerous because they cause cardiovascular problems.

c. All new diabetics must go on insulin first until they are stabilized.

d. Insulin may be able to cure diabetes for you.

150. An 86-year-old woman was admitted to the critical care unit after a fall that resulted in a subdural hematoma. The most important risk to watch for during her acute care hospital stay is:

a. Changes in BUN and creatinine levels, indicating renal failure

b. Rise in triglyceride levels

c. Effect of altered sensation on nutrition status

d. Onset of delirium

151. The study of the actions and effects of drugs is:

a. Pharmacokinetics

b. Pharmacology

c. Pharmacodynamics

d. Pharmacogenomics

152. An older patient complains of sudden blindness in his left eye. He says he has severe myopia, wears his glasses, and has never experienced anything like this. He notes that he was golfing in the morning and rode in a golf cart over a very bumpy course. This is a vision-threatened situation requiring immediate treatment by an ophthalmologist because it is:

    a. Wet macular degeneration

    b. Detached retina

    c. Dry macular degeneration

    d. Acute angle glaucoma

153. A hallmark(s) of palliative care is:

    a. Creating a peaceful environment

    b. Management of psychological symptoms such as anxiety and depression

    c. Good communication among the interdisciplinary team, patient, and family

    d. All of the above

154. Pneumonia is a common reason for hospital admission for older adults. People with weakened immune systems, rusty sputum, and productive cough are more likely to experience which infection:

    a. *Streptococcus pneumoniae*

    b. *Haemophilus influenzae*

    c. *Staphylococcus aureus*

    d. *Klebsiella pneumoniae*

155. In discussing sexually transmitted infections (STIs) with older adults, nurses should know that:

    a. Protection against STIs is not an important part of older adult's lives.

    b. Impotency is a natural occurrence with age.

    c. Condoms may be used to protect older adults against STIs.

    d. Men older than 75 years of age are incapable of fathering a child.

156. Symptoms of macular degeneration include:

    a. Floaters and blind spots

    b. Blurred vision and difficulty reading

    c. Blind spots and diplopia

    d. Trouble with night vision and astigmatism

157. When assessing laboratory results, a nurse sees that the blood cholesterol level of a newly admitted patient is over 240 mg/dL. This finding indicates that this patient has a:

    a. Desirable blood cholesterol level

    b. Borderline blood cholesterol level

    c. High blood cholesterol level

    d. Critical blood cholesterol level

158. A respiratory assessment of an older adult should include which of the following?

    a. Inspection, palpation, and auscultation

    b. Inspection and auscultation

    c. Inspection, palpation, percussion, and auscultation

    d. Palpation and auscultation

159. Because the presentation of an acute myocardial infarction in an older patient is atypical, it is important to monitor older patients carefully when they complain of which of the following?

    a. Shortness of breath, leg cramps, or headache

    b. Proximal extremity pain, dizziness, or chest pain

    c. Shortness of breath, fatigue, or epigastric discomfort

    d. Chest pain, headache, or tingling in proximal extremities

160. You are interviewing Mr. L, who has a hearing impairment. What techniques would be most beneficial in communicating with him?

    a. Request a sign language interpreter before you meet with Mr. L to facilitate the communication.

    b. Speak loudly and with exaggerated facial movements when talking with Mr. L, because this helps with lip reading.

    c. Avoid using facial and hand gestures, because most hearing-impaired people find this degrading.

    d. Assess Mr. L's preferred method of communication.

161. Disengagement is an example of what type of theory of aging?

    a. Biological

    b. Sociological

    c. Psychological

    d. Moral/spiritual

162. The Five Rights of Delegation was developed by which nursing organization?

    a. American Nurses Association

    b. National League for Nursing

    c. American Association of Critical Care Nurses

    d. National Council of State Boards of Nursing

163. Sleep complaints among older adults commonly involve which of the following?

    a. Difficulty falling asleep

    b. Frequent nighttime awakenings

    c. Both a and b

    d. None of the above

164. An 86-year-old man was admitted to the critical care unit and is now exhibiting signs of delirium. It is important to explain to concerned family members that delirium _____ that is often caused by _____ in the hospitalized elderly.

    a. Is reversible/medications

    b. Is irreversible/chronic obstructive pulmonary disease (COPD)

    c. Is part of the normal aging process/stress

    d. Develops over a long period of time/genetic factors

165. In gerontological nursing, all of the following are good examples of rehabilitative care, *except:*

    a. The process of assisting disabled persons to return to optimal health

    b. A specialized type of care that assists older adults to reach maximum functional capacity physically, mentally, and emotionally

    c. A type of care that restores the older person to a healthful state

    d. A low-level type of care in which the emphasis is on doing to the patient rather than working with the patient

166. Because of the tendency among older adults to experience folic acid deficiency anemia, nurses need to teach older adults to eat a diet rich in:

    a. Salmon, tuna, and walnuts

    b. Nuts, liver, and green leafy vegetables

    c. Apples, pears, and strawberries

    d. Legumes, cereal, and dairy foods

167. To provide best-practice health care to older adults, it is necessary to assess and measure quality care indicators. Most institutions have which of the following committees measure the data?

  a. Ethics

  b. Quality improvement

  c. Safety

  d. Risk monitoring

168. An 81-year-old man has recurrent arthritic inflammation of several peripheral joints. He was diagnosed with gout 2 years ago and asks you to explain what causes this inflammation. You explain that:

  a. "When you have an infection, your body secretes uric acid, which triggers the inflammation."

  b. "Because you also have osteoarthritis, you are at risk for more inflammation from the joints, and this causes the gout."

  c. "You have excess uric acid, which creates deposits of urate crystals in the soft tissue surrounding your peripheral joints."

  d. "The inflammation is triggered by heat and physical activity."

169. Cognitive status needs to be assessed when older adults present with acute illnesses because their cognitive ability may be temporarily affected by the illness. This acute change in cognitive status is termed:

  a. Dementia

  b. Confusion

  c. Delirium

  d. Agitation

170. Physical restraints should only be used under the most severe circumstances. If physical restraints are used, which of the following interventions are necessary?

  a. Check the restraints once every 8 hours.

  b. Keep restraints on a minimum of 3 days.

  c. Document why restraints are ordered, how they will be evaluated, and when they should be discontinued.

  d. Release the restraints at least every 4 hours, and move the restrained body part through full range of motion.

171. A 79-year-old woman returns to the nursing home with her daughter after attending a seafood chowder dinner. She complains of itching in her throat, a slightly swollen tongue, and mild shortness of breath. What is she experiencing?

    a. Allergic rhinitis

    b. Drug interaction

    c. Anaphylaxis

    d. Cerebrovascular accident

172. Which of the following interventions would a nurse include in the care plan of a patient with a pressure ulcer?

    a. Apply pressure to boney prominences.

    b. Check areas at risk every 10 minutes.

    c. Avoid cushion devices that prevent pressure ulcers on the coccyx.

    d. Turn and reposition the patient every 1 to 2 hours.

173. A research tool that has validity indicates:

    a. A strong probability that it has been standardized in this country

    b. The tool measures what it is intended to measure

    c. The data have been randomly collected

    d. The findings are reliable

174. Nurses need to know that stress incontinence:

    a. Can be caused by bladder muscle weakness

    b. Is also called neurogenic bladder

    c. Is a leakage of urine resulting from weakened deltoid muscles

    d. Results in the total uncontrolled and continuous loss of urine

175. A 68-year-old man has been diagnosed with Parkinson's disease. He is on several medications to manage his movement disorders that include:

    a. Rigidity, bradykinesia, and tremors

    b. Tremors, incontinence, and aphasia

    c. Gait problems, salivation, and aphasia

    d. Seizures, rigidity, and balance

176. One attempt to address the health care needs of U.S. citizens, especially those in long-term care settings, occurred as a result of which governmental act?

    a. Social Security Act

    b. Omnibus Budget Reconciliation Act

    c. Racketeer Influence Corrupt Organization Act

    d. Soldiers and Sailors Relief Act

177. A person who is malnourished may have reduced albumin levels, which cause levels of free drugs to:

    a. Decrease

    b. Bind to sodium

    c. Increase

    d. Bind to calcium

178. Physical changes in older women that affect sexual activity include:

    a. Enlargement of the breast

    b. Increased lubrication of the vaginal mucosa

    c. Decrease in the production of estrogen

    d. Decrease in vaginal size

179. A 72-year-old man at the adult day care center where you work tells you that he has a dark mole on his back that appears to be growing. The best action would be to:

    a. Arrange an appointment for him to see the physician.

    b. Tell him to monitor the mole's growth rate for 5 to 6 months.

    c. Have him come to the center for a weekly check of the mole.

    d. Tell him not to worry, because most moles are not a serious medical condition.

180. Older adults are expected to represent what percentage of the population by the year 2030?

    a. 0%

    b. 13%

    c. 21%

    d. 45%

181. Older adults who experience urinary tract infections (UTIs) can sometimes present with which of the following *atypical* symptoms?

    a. Dysuria

    b. Pain in the pubic area

    c. Confusion

    d. Flank pain

182. An 82-year-old woman's husband has recently died, and she has been preparing to move from her home to her daughter's home. She notices she has a linear papular rash on the left side of her spine that is very painful. This is most likely:

    a. Herpes simplex 1 virus

    b. Herpes zoster

    c. Herpes simplex 2 virus

    d. Herpes virus 8

183. An 82-year-old woman is diagnosed with glaucoma and prescribed timolol ophthalmic solution (Timoptic), 1 drop in her right eye twice a day. She is already taking metoprolol (Toprol-XL), 100 mg every day for hypertension. It is important to emphasize that she should notify you if she experiences which of the following?

    a. Dizziness

    b. Headache

    c. Visual changes

    d. Weakness

184. It is important for nurse managers to make decisions regarding health care delivery costs by using a:

    a. Cost–benefit analysis

    b. Mean ratio of what is necessary for best practice

    c. Cost–utility analysis

    d. None of the above

185. Restraints may come in all of the following forms, *except:*

    a. Side rails

    b. Vests

    c. Pharmacological

    d. Restorative

186. Mr. Brown, newly admitted to your nursing home, approaches you complaining of constipation. You explain to him that this is a common occurence in aging because of all of the following reasons, *except:*

    a. Lack of privacy

    b. Altered cognitive status

    c. Decreased bulk in the diet

    d. Decreased bowel peristalsis

187. Which symptom would be most characteristic of a UTI?

    a. Fever greater than 102°F

    b. Sharp pain in the abdomen

    c. Pain and discomfort when urinating

    d. Inability to void

188. An important factor to assess in the history-taking component of a physical exam is:

    a. Appointments the patient may have made at other medical facilities

    b. Drug allergies

    c. Whether the person has a pet

    d. Recent experience with fast-food services

189. Due to the effect of inhibition of norepinephrine and serotonin reuptake by tramadol, it is not recommended for older adults who have a:

    a. History of seizures

    b. Concurrent use of steroids

    c. History of diabetes mellitus

    d. Concurrent use of diuretics

190. A 71-year-old woman has Parkinson's disease and is asking what the etiology of her illness is. You would include which of the following?

    a. Disorder of movement caused by cerebellar disease

    b. Disorder of the substantia nigra that decreases ability to initiate movement

    c. Brain disorder caused by aging that decreases beta cells

    d. Disorder of the pons that creates excessive cerebrospinal fluid in the brain

191. Neuropathic pain, such as that experienced in postherpetic neuralgia, is common among older adults. Which of the following drug categories is frequently used for treatment of neuropathic pain?

    a. Anticonvulsants

    b. Opiates

    c. NSAIDs

    d. Acetaminophen (Tylenol)

192. A physiological change due to aging that affects gas exchange in the respiratory system is:

    a. Increased carbon monoxide excretion

    b. Decreased carbon anion movement at the capillary membrane

    c. Decreased passage of oxygen from the alveoli to the blood

    d. Increased oxygen binding capacity for hemoglobin

193. The main function of a mentor for a professional nurse is to:

    a. Assist with career goal accomplishment

    b. Work side by side on patient care

    c. Become a good friend

    d. Demonstrate complex clinical interventions

194. The scope of practice that a nurse can exercise is determined by the:

    a. State's Nurse Practice Act

    b. Federal government

    c. American Nurses Association

    d. State government

195. Many older people have itchy, dry skin. Which are the best interventions to remedy this situation?

    a. Use less soap because it is drying, keep well hydrated, apply emollient cream

    b. Bathe more frequently, drink high-sodium beverages, use sunscreen

    c. Keep well hydrated, take frequent oatmeal baths, apply mineral oil

    d. Restrict time in sun, use sunscreen, wear light cotton clothing

196. Approximately what percentage of older adults is noncompliant with health care treatment plans?

    a. 25%

    b. 50%

    c. 75%

    d. 100%

197. A 72-year-old woman is admitted with pedal edema, rales, shortness of breath, confusion, and recent weight gain. She has a history of well-controlled hypertension but no history of chest pain. She most likely will be diagnosed with which of the following leading reasons for hospitalization for older adults?

    a. Hypertension

    b. Heart failure

    c. Coronary artery disease

    d. Myocardial infarction

198. Mr. Jackson needs to leave his own home for an alternative residence. The reasons that older adults move from one environment to another include all of the following, *except:*

    a. Increased income

    b. Onset of illness

    c. Change in family dynamics

    d. Insufficient funds to maintain home

199. Gerotranscendence is an example of what type of theory of aging?

    a. Biological

    b. Pathological

    c. Physiological

    d. Psychosocial

200. A few weeks after admission to a rehabilitation facility, Mr. Violet developed sudden onset of cognitive changes. You would most likely suspect which of the following?

    a. UTI

    b. Peripheral vascular disease

    c. Malignant growth of a previously benign tumor

    d. Gynecomastia

201. Pressure ulcers generally occur over which part of the body?

    a. Spine

    b. Toes

    c. Bony prominences

    d. Knees

202. After an older adult falls, it is customary to perform an assessment that would include which of the following?

    a. Cognitive, psychological, and neurological assessments

    b. Focused physical exam and functional assessment

    c. Focused history and physical exam as well as a review of functional ability and medications

    d. Incident report and notification of patient's lawyer

203. Due to the shrinking of the thymus gland with aging, older adults are more prone for infections due to:

    a. Increased hypersensitivity response

    b. Diminished T cell responsiveness

    c. Secondary antibody response

    d. Increase in antibody formation

204. Many older men experience fungal infection of their toenails. Symptoms such as thickened, distorted, and yellowish color indicate:

    a. Tinea pedis

    b. Tinea versicolor

    c. Onychomycosis

    d. Balanitis

205. Regarding the sleep patterns of older adults, nurses should know that:

    a. Older adults are more tolerant to shifts in the sleep–wake cycle.

    b. Daytime napping of many older adults seems to compensate for nighttime sleep disturbances.

    c. Rapid-eye-movement sleep increases with age.

    d. Older adults have a higher quality of sleep than younger adults.

206. In nursing research, a placebo intervention is generally used for the:

 a. Experimental group

 b. Control group

 c. Variant group

 d. Testing group

207. Lipid deposits in the eyes of some older adults are manifested by:

 a. A bluish circle on the aqueous humor

 b. A grayish arc surrounding the cornea

 c. Drusen bodies (yellow pigment) in the macula

 d. Cotton balls in the retina

208. A type of health care insurance for older adults that is funded and regulated by the federal government is called:

 a. Medicare

 b. Medicaid

 c. Private insurance

 d. Medigap

209. Glomerular filtration decreases as a result of aging, and it can be further decreased by:

 a. Increased blood flow to the kidneys

 b. Some medications

 c. Penicillin sensitivity

 d. Stress

210. Older adults experience a decrease in taste sensation. Which of the following factors can further decrease the sense of taste?

 a. Diabetes, medications, dehydration

 b. Medications, fatigue, oral ulcers

 c. Infections, smoking, medications

 d. Medications, poor dentition, dehydration

211. What is the greatest risk factor for a fall?

 a. Age

 b. Cognitive impairment

 c. Osteoporosis

 d. Previous history of a fall

212. Gerontological nurses should advise patients with degenerative osteoarthritis to:

   a. Rest the involved joints as much as possible.

   b. Apply ice to the painful joints.

   c. Apply heat to the painful joints.

   d. Exercise the involved joints regularly.

213. The Patient's Bill of Rights mandates that each patient in a long-term care facility or hospital has the right to:

   a. Information disclosure, access to emergency services, and participation in treatment decisions

   b. Access to his or her medications, dietary choice, and participation in treatment decisions

   c. Information disclosure, the right to choose one's roommate, and a translator

   d. A translator, access to emergency service, and dietary choice

214. A 68-year-old man has experienced GERD for many years and has managed it with daily omeprazole (Prilosec). He has a hiatal hernia repair, and his physician suggests that an additional test be done while he is hospitalized. Most likely, this test is to assess for:

   a. Gastric acid contents

   b. Intrinsic acid depletion

   c. *Helicobacter pylori*

   d. Diverticulosis

215. A 68-year-old patient is prediabetic with a fasting blood sugar of 108. As the visiting nurse performing his wound care, you teach him about how important which of the following activities are to promote his health and possibly prevent his being diagnosed with diabetes in the future?

   a. Exercising regularly every day, losing weight, stopping smoking

   b. Taking insulin, eating a low-salt diet, stopping smoking

   c. Avoiding stress, eating a diet high in omega fats

   d. Joining a palliative care support group, eating a low-carbohydrate diet

216. When assessing an older adult's mobility and overall function, the timed Up and Go test is quite comprehensive and a normal result should only take about:

  a. 2 minutes

  b. 1 minute

  c. 30 seconds

  d. 10 seconds

217. A nursing home patient is complaining of increased thirst and a dry mouth. You are not surprised to see that she is on:

  a. Bupropion hydrochloride (Wellbutrin)

  b. Oxybutynin (Ditropan)

  c. Furosemide (Lasix)

  d. Spironolactone (Aldactone)

218. A 67-year-old woman has Raynaud's syndrome. She complains of cold fingers intermittently throughout the year. She has trouble doing her needlepoint and asks if there is any medication she can take to "warm up her fingers." Your response is:

  a. "There are vasodilators that could be used, but they may cause too much constriction in other vessels."

  b. "Have you tried wearing gloves when your fingers get cold?"

  c. "Let's discuss this with the physician next month when she comes for your physical exam."

  d. "There are medications that would dilate the small vessels in your hands and fingers, but these drugs would dilate other vessels, too, which could cause harm."

219. It is paramount to follow the Institute of Medicine's guidelines in order to improve:

  a. Staff retention

  b. The safety culture of the institution

  c. Medical and nursing malpractice insurance coverage

  d. Nurse satisfaction

220. A woman accompanies her mother to the clinic. She tells the nurse that her mother has been experiencing recent memory loss. The nurse should first assess the mother's:

    a. Cognitive status

    b. Dietary status

    c. Temperature

    d. Ability to ambulate

221. One rationale supporting the idea that aging causes people to become shorter is:

    a. Weakened vertebrae cause disk compression

    b. Increased osteoblast activity

    c. Decreased osteoclast activity

    d. Increased estrogen levels

222. Mrs. Goldberg is nearing the end of her life and has ordered hospice care. The focus of hospice care is:

    a. Restorative

    b. Rehabilitative

    c. Palliative

    d. Curative

223. Advance directives are designed to:

    a. Provide details about a patient's estate after death.

    b. Provide information on who should get the patient's car after death.

    c. Provide information on the patient's wishes after death.

    d. Provide information on a patient's wishes at the end of life.

224. Which of the following agencies accredit facilities such as long-term care agencies?

    a. Safety Coalition

    b. Joint Commission of Hospital Accrediting Organization

    c. The Joint Commission

    d. Older American Services Bureau

225. Which of the following assessment findings is most important to report when caring for an elderly patient with heart failure?

   a. The patient develops confusion or exhibits a change in mental status.

   b. The patient's blood pressure is 110/60.

   c. The patient's weight is unchanged.

   d. The patient complains of a headache.

226. Good nutrition is an example of which type of prevention?

   a. Primary

   b. Secondary

   c. Tertiary

   d. Preventative

227. Hayflick theory is an example of what type of theory of aging?

   a. Biological

   b. Sociological

   c. Psychological

   d. Moral/spiritual

228. An 81-year-old woman has her annual exam, and the blood work reveals increased serum iron ferritin, decreased iron, and decreased total iron-binding capacity. You are not surprised, because this woman receives which of the following treatments?

   a. Renal dialysis every other day

   b. Physical therapy daily

   c. Speech articulation therapy weekly

   d. Hydrotherapy for hips daily

229. Most older adults with hypertension are not prescribed antihypertensive drugs from which of the following categories because of decreased beta receptor sensitivity in the elderly?

   a. Calcium channel blockers

   b. Diuretics

   c. Beta blockers

   d. Alpha blockers

230. Which assessment tool has been used in assessing functional status in older adults?

    a. Beers Criteria

    b. Maslow Guidelines

    c. Katz Index

    d. Mini-Mental State Exam

231. With orthostatic hypotension in older adults, it is important to assess for which of the following symptoms after a position change?

    a. Palpitations and headache

    b. Dizziness and palpitations

    c. Dizziness and lightheadedness

    d. Lightheadedness and palpitations

232. A type of health care insurance for older adults that is funded and regulated by the state government is called:

    a. Medicare

    b. Medicaid

    c. Private insurance

    d. Medigap

233. A 77-year-old man complains of not being able to hear well. He denies any problems with tinnitus or ear pain. He most likely is experiencing:

    a. Perforated tympanic membrane

    b. Otitis externa

    c. Otitis media

    d. Cerumen impaction

234. Which of the following joints endure the most impact from osteoarthritis and need to be assessed carefully?

    a. Ankles and fibulas

    b. Large toe and ankle joints

    c. Tibias and ankles

    d. Hips and knees

235. Many older adults experience problems with their feet due to poorly fitting shoes. The condition that results from pressure from a shoe rubbing against the bony areas of the toes is:

    a. Bunion

    b. Corn

    c. Hallux valgus

    d. Callus

236. A gerontological nurse is researching symptom management in palliative care for older adults in long-term care facilities. The purpose of the study is to collect specific information over a period of 6 months about the number of pain medication interventions and level of distress (on a 0–10 scale) from pain. Which method of research should be used to collect data?

    a. Qualitative research

    b. Interviewing of patient families' perceptions

    c. Quantitative research

    d. Delphi survey

237. A 70-year-old woman complains of a lump on her neck in her thyroid gland. She is admitted to the hospital for diagnostic testing that will include:

    a. Fine-needle biopsy

    b. X-ray of thyroid

    c. CT scan of neck

    d. MRI of upper body

238. Hospitals are required to:

    a. Write advance directives on all patients.

    b. Make sure patients develop advance directives before surgery.

    c. Provide patients the opportunity to develop advance directives.

    d. File advance directives in medical records room immediately upon admission.

239. One of the main causes of delirium is:

    a. Age

    b. COPD

    c. Medications

    d. Participation in treatment decision making

240. Many older adults deny that they have pain and try to maintain their routine without taking medications for pain. Which of the following sets of words may assist in obtaining more accurate pain assessment?

    a. Visual analogue scale of 0 to 10, asking them to point to their pain, asking them to explain their concerns

    b. Discomfort, hurting, aching

    c. Nociceptive pain, neuropathic pain, mixed pain sensation

    d. Autonomic, sympathetic, parasympathetic

241. Immunization is an example of which type of prevention?

    a. Primary

    b. Secondary

    c. Tertiary

    d. Preventative

242. Due to the aging process, it is not appropriate to use skin turgor as an indicator of fluid status; rather, one would use which of the following parameters to assess dehydration in older patients?

    a. Intake and output, mucous membrane moisture, and urine specific gravity

    b. Volume of respiratory secretions, intake and output, capillary refill

    c. Intake and output, mental status, and jugular venous distention

    d. Urine specific gravity, thirst, and intake and output

243. Durable power of attorney provides which information if a patient should experience a terminal condition or a permanent state of unconsciousness?

    a. Written information describing desires for life-sustaining treatment

    b. Names a person for making health care decisions

    c. Provides information for the distribution of financial assets

    d. Provides for terminal care at the end of life

244. Mrs. B, 75 years old, is at your clinic for a preoperative interview. This interview may take longer than an interview with a younger patient because:

    a. As people age, they are unable to hear and thus interviewers need to repeat much more of what is said.

    b. Older people lose much of their mental capacity and require more time to complete an interview.

c. An older person has a longer story to tell.

d. An older person is usually lonely and likes to have someone to talk to.

245. Self-actualization is an example of what type of theory of aging?

a. Biological

b. Sociological

c. Psychological

d. Moral/spiritual

246. As one ages, estrogen decreases and negatively influences bone growth by:

a. Increasing osteoblast function

b. Decreasing osteoblast function

c. Decreasing osteoclast function

d. Balancing calcitonin release

247. Immunosenescence refers to the aging of the immunological system and primarily affects which of the following in older adults?

a. B cells

b. CD_{12} cells

c. T cells

d. Hepatocyte cells

248. The prescription and administration of more medications than are clinically appropriate for an individual is often seen with older adults. This is called:

a. Pharmacogenesis

b. Drug toxicity

c. Polypharmacy

d. Overdose

249. Due to a smaller number of functioning cilia and a less effective cough in older adults, there is more potential for acute respiratory infections to progress to:

a. Pulmonary edema

b. Pleural effusion

c. Pneumonia

d. Pneumothorax

250. An 84-year-old patient is experiencing cramp-like pain in his abdomen that awakens him from his sleep and is relieved with food ingestion. He says he has had this before for about 2 weeks at a time, and then it disappears. He most likely has:

    a. A gastric ulcer

    b. A duodenal ulcer

    c. Gastritis

    d. Crohn's disease

251. The nursing administration at a long-term care facility wants to assess patient and family perceptions of their facility's ability to manage patients' pain. They are interested in determining what the patients and families like about the current process and what they would like to change. To conduct this study, they will use a focus group. A focus group is an example of which type of research?

    a. Quantitative research

    b. Qualitative research

    c. Experimental research

    d. Gerontological standard survey

252. Problems with the U.S. health care system have stimulated many attempts at health care reform. Diagnostic related groups created in the 1980s attempted to correct which major problem of the health care delivery system?

    a. Poor care provided by hospitals

    b. Poor care provided by home care agencies

    c. Poor care in mental institutions

    d. Rising Medicare costs

253. Because of the multiple side effects of various medications, most older adults have most effective pain relief with the fewest side effects by taking:

    a. Propoxyphene

    b. Acetaminophen (Tylenol)

    c. Meperidine (Demerol)

    d. Pentazocine

254. A treatment option for depression that blocks the reabsorption of serotonin is:

    a. Elavil

    b. Zoloft

    c. Haldol

    d. Restoril

255. A healthy older adult may manifest all the following changes in the respiratory system, *except:*

    a. Thoracic cage stiffening

    b. Decreased cough

    c. Fewer alveoli

    d. Fewer cilia

256. PSA testing is an example of which type of prevention?

    a. Primary

    b. Secondary

    c. Tertiary

    d. Preventative

257. A few weeks after admission to a long-term care facility, an 84-year-old female developed sudden-onset cognitive changes. You would most likely suspect which of the following?

    a. UTI

    b. Peripheral vascular disease

    c. Malignant growth of a previously benign tumor

    d. Gynecomastia

258. Activity theory is an example of what type of theory of aging?

    a. Biological

    b. Sociological

    c. Psychological

    d. Moral/spiritual

259. Which are some of the side effects of opioids that can impact the functional ability of older adults?

    a. Increased appetite, need for increased hydration, increased libido

    b. Gait disturbance, dizziness, impaired concentration

    c. Abdominal fullness, thirst, hunger

    d. Diarrhea, dry mouth, hunger

260. The hospice philosophy of care affirms the patient's right to:

    a. Live and die with dignity

    b. Pain management while maintaining mental alertness

    c. A confusion-free end of life

    d. Spiritual wholeness

261. Benign prostatic hyperplasia occurs in approximately 50% of men by age 65. Common symptoms include which of the following?

    a. Flatus, abdominal distention, bladder fullness

    b. Polyuria, urinary urgency, increased frequency

    c. Dysuria, nocturia, bladder spasm

    d. Bladder fullness, dysuria, polyuria

262. It can be difficult to perform physical examinations of older adults for all of the following reasons, *except:*

    a. Polypharmacy

    b. Lack of standards

    c. Presbyopia

    d. Normal aging changes

263. Change theory recommends that nurse managers will be most successful in making a change if:

    a. The entire staff is involved in any decision making regarding the change.

    b. The nurses most interested in making the change are involved.

    c. Only the nurse manager controls the change implementation.

    d. The entire staff evaluates the outcomes of the change.

264. Consequences of persistent pain with older adults include:

    a. Headache, metallic taste, abdominal fullness

    b. Lower extremity cramping, bladder fullness, infection

    c. Flat affect, diarrhea, spasticity of bowel

    d. Depression, anxiety, sleep disturbance

265. A 72-year-old woman has shingles and is expecting to have visitors today, among them her pregnant niece. She should be instructed not to have contact with the following individuals:

    a. Pregnant women, infants, people who are immunocompromised

    b. People who have diabetes, vaccinated school-age children, infants

    c. People who did not have chicken pox, older adults, people who have diabetes

    d. People with tuberculosis, mononucleosis, or liver failure

266. A 66-year-old woman admitted to the hospital for a sudden headache— "the worst headache of my life"—is diagnosed with a subarachnoid hemorrhage. What would her manifestations include?

    a. Headache, seizures, vomiting

    b. Seizures, change in sense of smell and taste

    c. Headache, stiff neck, hypotension

    d. Photophobia, headache, diplopia

267. Mrs. Jasmine is complaining of problems sleeping and requests a sleep agent. Which of the following medications would be unsafe to give her?

    a. Ambien

    b. Benadryl

    c. Halcion

    d. Midularium

268. Mrs. Carlson, a 73-year-old woman newly admitted to your nursing home, has a score on a GDS indicating that she has depression. Your first line of treatment for her would be to:

    a. Refer her for psychotherapy.

    b. Recommend to her physician the need for immediate antidepressant medication.

    c. Do nothing, because this is a normal change of aging.

    d. Arrange a psychiatric consult for evaluation of her depression and treatment.

269. The hospice philosophy supports that dying is:
    a. Almost always preventable
    b. A natural part of life
    c. Often associated with pain
    d. Best supported with intensive care

270. Who is the nurse theorist associated with the concept of adaptation?
    a. Sister Callista Roy
    b. Jean Watson
    c. Martha Rogers
    d. Imogene M. King

271. Cholesterol screening is an example of which type of prevention?
    a. Primary
    b. Secondary
    c. Tertiary
    d. Preventative

272. Medicare typically pays what percentage of the usual customary and reasonable rate?
    a. 20%
    b. 50%
    c. 80%
    d. 100%

273. The inability of a caregiver to identify and provide for needs among older adults is classified as which type of elder mistreatment?
    a. Physical
    b. Psychological
    c. Active neglect
    d. Passive neglect

274. A couple in their 80s have been experiencing problems tasting their food and request information regarding this. After giving them several ideas, you specifically mention alternatives to improve which of the following taste sensations that particularly tend to decrease with aging?
    a. Salt and sugar
    b. All types of beef
    c. Lemon and other citrus fruits
    d. Tartness

275. An 88-year-old man complains of dizziness when getting into bed from his wheelchair and getting into his wheelchair from his bed. It is important for the nurse to assess for orthostatic hypotension on this patient. The nurse should test the man's:

    a. Blood pressure and pulse while lying, sitting, and standing

    b. Blood pressure while lying, sitting, and standing

    c. Blood pressure in his right and left arms while sitting

    d. Blood pressure upon awakening and immediately before he changes position

276. After hip replacement for a hip fracture, patients are taught to maintain abduction. Thus, these patients are told not to cross their legs because it may cause:

    a. Dislocation of the prosthesis

    b. Subluxation of the hip

    c. Incomplete dislocation of the joint

    d. Angular alignment

277. You are bathing an 80-year-old man and notice that his skin is wrinkled, thin, lax, and dry. This finding is related to which normal change of aging?

    a. Integumentary system changes

    b. Increases in elastin and subcutaneous fat

    c. An increase in the number of sweat and sebaceous glands

    d. Increased vascular flow to the skin

278. When does a geriatric nurse's work with dying clients end?

    a. When the patient dies.

    b. When the patient is in a pain-free state.

    c. When the patient reaches self-actualization.

    d. When the family's grieving process is complete.

279. Mr. Paul was admitted to your medical–surgical unit after a radical prostatectomy. He has been yelling and trying to remove his IV. The reason for his behavior is most likely:

    a. Dementia

    b. Delirium

    c. Depression

    d. Bipolar disease

280. A 66-year-old woman has osteopenia. Which of the following drugs is likely to be prescribed to inhibit osteoclast activity and increase bone mass?

   a. Fluoride

   b. Risedronate (Actonel)

   c. Parathyroid hormone

   d. Estrogen replacement

281. For an elderly patient who was prescribed nitroglycerin to be left at the bedside for self-administration, it would be important for the nurse to assess the patient's:

   a. Skin turgor

   b. Mental status for confusion or disorientation

   c. Ability to ambulate

   d. Past medical history

282. Orthostatic hypotension in older adults is diagnosed in which of the following situations?

   a. Systolic and diastolic blood pressure decreases of 10 mmHg after a position change

   b. Systolic blood pressure decrease of 20 mmHg and a diastolic blood pressure decrease of 10 mmHg after a position change

   c. Systolic and diastolic blood pressure decrease of 20 mmHg after a position change

   d. Systolic blood pressure decrease of 10 mmHg and diastolic blood pressure decrease of 20 mmHg after a position change

283. Gerontological nurses follow the *Code of Ethics for Nurses* in their daily practice. These codes were developed by the:

   a. National League for Nursing

   b. American Geriatrics Society

   c. American Nurses Association

   d. State Board of Nursing

284. As men age, they experience _____ in erectile function as part of the normal aging process.

   a. An increase

   b. An improvement

   c. A decline

   d. A loss

285. A healthy older adult may manifest all the following skin changes, *except:*
    a. Decrease and thinning of body hair
    b. Increased facial hair in women
    c. Fingernails becoming more brittle
    d. Balding in patches

286. A client at an adult day care center asked the nurse about the term *presbycusis*. The nurse told the client that presbycusis:
    a. Is a sensorineural hearing loss that usually occurs bilaterally
    b. Is a progressive conductive hearing loss that commonly occurs with age
    c. Affects more women than men
    d. Is a type of hearing loss related to the administration of medication that is toxic to the organs of hearing

287. An 83-year-old man was diagnosed with a hiatal hernia. He had several symptoms similar to those caused by GERD, which included:
    a. Heartburn after a big meal or when lying supine
    b. Chest pain radiating to the left arm and shoulder
    c. Upper sternal pain immediately after a meal
    d. Right-sided chest pain on inspiration

288. Mr. Carter states that he is concerned because he notices a light-colored ring around the iris of his eye. What is the most appropriate response by the nurse?
    a. Tell Mr. Carter to talk to the physician about these types of concerns.
    b. Report this information to the charge nurse.
    c. Explain to Mr. Carter that this is a normal age-related change that occurs in the eye.
    d. Tell Mr. Carter that this condition could cause complications and must be monitored closely.

289. The most common type of incontinence that occurs with aging is _____ and is easily treated with _____.
    a. Overflow/bladder training
    b. Stress/Kegel exercises
    c. Transient/medication
    d. Urge/surgery

290. Geriatric nurses may best assist a grieving family by:
    a. Using an active listening approach to communication
    b. Stating that the patient died a "good death"
    c. Encouraging an expeditious burial
    d. Sharing in-depth details about his or her own experiences with a dying relative

291. Active listening incorporates several techniques, such as:
    a. Open questioning, accommodation, and collaboration
    b. Conflict management, acknowledging, and negotiating
    c. Open questioning, acknowledging, and summarizing
    d. Framing, grouping similar ideas, and accommodation

292. Who was the founder of hospice?
    a. Ada Sue Hinshaw
    b. Adelaide Nutting
    c. Victoria Champion
    d. Dame Cicely Saunders

293. Who is the nurse theorist associated with the concept of self-care?
    a. Florence Nightingale
    b. Virginia Henderson
    c. Martha Rogers
    d. Dorothea Orem

294. It is important to realize that older adults with acute respiratory failure present a challenge for health management due to their:
    a. Increased work of breathing, increased compliance, increased $PaCO_2$
    b. Lifelong smoking habit, cardiovascular disease, increased vital capacity
    c. Decreased respiratory muscle strength, decreased airway and lung compliance
    d. Increased vital capacity, comorbidities, decreased work of breathing

295. Neurologic cell changes that occur with aging include a deposition of Lewy bodies that are linked with a specific type of

    a. Obesity

    b. Heart failure

    c. Dementia

    d. Depression

296. Speech pathology is an example of which type of prevention?

    a. Primary

    b. Secondary

    c. Tertiary

    d. Preventative

297. Hospital insurance for Medicare recipients is funded under:

    a. Medicare Part A

    b. Medicaid Part A

    c. Medicare Part B

    d. Medicaid Part B

298. An age-related change of the musculoskeletal system is:

    a. Height decreases with age, and posture becomes straighter and more defined.

    b. The lengthening of the spinal column results in a dowager's hump.

    c. Muscle fibers shorten and increase in number.

    d. Bone reabsorption causes the bone to lose calcium and decreases the ability to produce material for the bone matrix.

299. There is an increase in the various forms of elder abuse and this is linked with an increase of older adults experiencing

    a. Posttraumatic stress disorder

    b. Obsessive-compulsive disorder

    c. Mania

    d. Schizophrenia

300. A 72-year-old man presented in the emergency department with left sternal pain radiating into his left shoulder whenever he moves his left arm. Pain developed over the past 3 days, after he had built a small fence in his yard. He denies palpitation, shortness of breath, or dyspnea on exertion. His laboratory parameters and electrocardiogram are within normal limits. His pain is most likely:

   a. Muscular pain from overuse

   b. Atypical chest pain

   c. Anginal equivalent

   d. Rotator cuff dislocation

301. Taking several medications is referred to as:

   a. Polypharmacy

   b. A drug idiosyncrasy

   c. Toxicity

   d. A cumulative drug effect

302. Nurses on a unit make it a priority to have their morning care and medications completed by 10:00 a.m. for all their patients. The staff is task oriented and concentrates only on morning care and medications; they delay other patient concerns until after lunch. The nurse manager on this unit practices:

   a. Trait leadership

   b. Situational leadership

   c. Transformational leadership

   d. Transactional leadership

303. Regarding age-related changes associated with excretion, nurses should know that:

   a. Age does not affect the excretion of drugs to any appreciable degree.

   b. When the kidneys are not functioning properly, drugs tend to remain in the bloodstream longer, increasing the risk of drug toxicity.

   c. Most drugs do not affect kidney functioning.

   d. The GFR in the kidneys increases with age, resulting in an increase in the excretion of drugs.

304. The ultimate goals of quality-improvement programs in health care provide:
    a. Cost savings, patient satisfaction, and staff retention
    b. Optimal patient outcomes, access to services, and cost-effectiveness
    c. Family satisfaction, optimal patient outcomes, and new technology
    d. Patient satisfaction, access to services, and telehealth services

305. Hospice care may take place in which environment of care?
    a. Home
    b. Nursing home
    c. Hospital
    d. All of the above

306. Which of the following is an age-related change that occurs in the gastrointestinal tract?
    a. Most people become edentulous (lose their teeth).
    b. There is a decreased incidence of hiatal hernia.
    c. There is an increased incidence of pertussis.
    d. The secretions of the salivary glands diminish.

307. The process by which a drug passes into the circulation for distribution throughout the body is called:
    a. Absorption
    b. Distribution
    c. Metabolism
    d. Excretion

308. A 76-year-old woman has been diagnosed with bilateral age-related macular degeneration. Her main complaint is:
    a. Peripheral vision loss
    b. Eye pain
    c. Central vision loss
    d. Blind spot

309. A 78-year-old diagnosed with myelodysplastic syndrome for the past 2 years is admitted to the hospital because he is experiencing pancytopenia. This indicates he has:

    a. Anemia, leukemia, and non-Hodgkin's lymphoma

    b. Neutropenia, tuberculosis, and lupus erythematosus

    c. Neutropenia, anemia, and thrombocytopenia

    d. Thrombocytopenia, iron loss, and uveitis

310. A nurse assistant asks the nurse to explain the word *pharmacokinetics*. The nurse defines pharmacokinetics as:

    a. The action of drugs within the body

    b. The movement of drugs within the body

    c. The use of drugs within the body

    d. Treatment of disease with medications

311. A 78-year-old woman has recently been diagnosed with chronic renal disease and is extremely fatigued. As the charge nurse, you communicate this to the medical director, who prescribes which of the following to assist in increasing red blood cells in the bone marrow?

    a. Ziagen (Abacavir)

    b. Stavudine (d4T)

    c. Erythropoietin (Epogen)

    d. Granulocyte colony-stimulating factor (Neupogen)

312. What information obtained in the health history would most likely have contributed to an older adult's COPD?

    a. Smoking since the age of 18

    b. Weight loss of 20 pounds in the past 6 months

    c. Working for 6 months as a construction worker

    d. No participation in a regular exercise program for the past several years

313. Which of the following theorists focused specifically on the nurse–patient interaction?

    a. Brenner and Wrubel

    b. Hildegard Peplau

    c. Madeleine Leininger

    d. Martha Rogers

314. The goal of nursing care at the end of life is to attain:

    a. Palliative care

    b. Good oral hygiene

    c. A "good death"

    d. As little pain as possible while maintaining alertness

315. A 76-year-old in a long-term care facility is working on a group quilting project. You notice she experiences tremors whenever she is sewing but no tremor when she is resting and waiting her turn. The tremor is most likely:

    a. Parkinsonian tremor

    b. Essential tremor

    c. Drug-induced tremor

    d. Vitamin-deficiency tremor

316. A 66-year-old woman takes an oral magnesium antacid regularly. Due to older adults' renal absorption, health teaching is necessary with this patient regarding the potential of getting:

    a. Hypokalemia

    b. Hypomagnesemia

    c. Hypermagnesemia

    d. Hypernatremia

317. The endocrine disease that is seen in both genders at a higher frequency than other adult-onset diseases is:

    a. Hyperthyroidism

    b. Hypothyroidism

    c. Hyperparathyroidism

    d. Hypoparathyroidism

318. Assessment of depression can be performed using which standardized tool specific for older adults?

    a. The GDS

    b. Beck's Anxiety and Depression Tool

    c. The Elderly Assessment of Depression

    d. The Suicide Assessment for Elders

319. Which of the following observations would a nurse expect to make in a patient with COPD?

    a. The patient has difficulty seeing distant objects.

    b. The patient complains of joint pain.

    c. The patient has difficulty falling asleep.

    d. The patient becomes short of breath when ambulating to the bathroom.

320. Older adults are more prone to developing type 2 diabetes mellitus due to:

    a. Decreased glucose intolerance

    b. Decreased sensitivity to insulin

    c. Increased glucose production

    d. Decreased insulin resistance

321. What is the CAGE questionnaire helpful in assessing?

    a. Readiness for smoking cessation

    b. Alcohol use

    c. Safe sex practices

    d. Amount of water drunk each day

322. After multiple admissions of patients to the nearby emergency department for worsening heart failure, the nurses at one long-term care facility decided to implement some new interventions to improve care for heart failure patients. They began by reviewing the literature regarding this topic and then adapted what they read. This practice model is known as:

    a. Evidence from the literature

    b. Evidence-based practice

    c. Content learned from others

    d. Knowledge-based research

323. Mrs. Lyons, 76 years old, has end-stage renal disease and is experiencing severe fatigue, is retaining fluid, and recently broke her wrist. These symptoms are due to:

    a. Increased circulating protein

    b. Electrolyte imbalance

    c. Lack of neutrophils

    d. Decreased granulocytes

324. Many older adults take medications, such as some of the statins, calcium channel blockers, and antiarrhythmics, and also enjoy eating grapefruit. It is important to teach these patients to follow this guideline:

    a. Stop eating grapefruit and drinking grapefruit juice.

    b. Take the medications 2 hours before eating grapefruit.

    c. Take the medications 2 hours after eating grapefruit.

    d. Eat grapefruit with the medications.

325. Due to pharmacokinetic changes in absorption, distribution, metabolism, and excretion of drugs with most older adults, there is increased:

    a. Metabolism of drugs

    b. Drug sensitivity

    c. Drug excretion

    d. Drug tolerance

326. Betty Jones, a 92-year-old woman, has just been admitted to your unit following a hip fracture. In planning her care, you are likely to consider the following points:

    a. Due to insurance regulations, Mrs. Jones will probably have a shorter length of stay than a younger patient would.

    b. Mrs. Jones will probably not be covered by Medicare.

    c. Mrs. Jones is probably confused.

    d. None of the above

327. A supercentenarian is:

    a. Someone living past 100, who is also free of disease

    b. Someone living past 110

    c. Someone living past 110, who is also free of disease

    d. Anyone over 120

328. Which of the following is true about the role of spirituality in aging?

    a. Faith practices tend to remain relatively stable over time.

    b. Most patients believe that it would not be appropriate to discuss matters of faith or spirituality in the health care setting.

    c. For most older adults, faith is a relatively minor way to cope with illness.

    d. As people age they become more religious.

329. Which of the following theories describes the theory that over time, DNA errors accumulate, eventually causing cell death?

    a. Stochastic

    b. Nonstochastic

    c. Nonphysiologic

    d. Damage theory

330. You are at home visiting your grandmother when something does not seem quite right. Her speech is slurred and one hand is hanging down. You decide to:

    a. Check her vital signs since you have your blood pressure cuff with you.

    b. Call her physician.

    c. Call 911.

    d. Recognize these as normal signs of aging.

331. You get a call that a friend of the family has had a stroke resulting in difficulty walking and speaking. The family wants to know what to expect next, you tell them:

    a. Older adults tend to stay in the hospital longer than young people do, so it is likely that he will be able to complete his recovery prior to discharge.

    b. He will likely need to go to a nursing home for rehabilitation.

    c. Poststroke recovery peaks 3 to 6 weeks following the event.

    d. You can expect a full recovery once the clot dissolves and the area of the brain is perfused again.

332. A group of nursing students conducts a small research project examining the most effective means to deliver medication education to older adults. Their sample consists of 100 adults from age 65 to 101 who live in the same community. The students conclude that individuals from age 65 to 101 prefer typewritten instructions. What is a potential problem with this study?

    a. The sample size of 100 is too small to draw any conclusions.

    b. The older adults ranging in age from 65 to 100+ were too diverse to be grouped into one category.

    c. It has been proved that older adults are not computer literate.

    d. The study design was not a randomized controlled trial.

333. When speaking to an older adult you should:

    a. Stand far away, to maintain a respectful distance.

    b. Show affection by using words of endearment like honey and sweetie.

    c. Speak softly and rapidly to communicate your ideas effectively.

    d. Address the older adult by his or her last name until instructed to do otherwise.

334. Which of the following statements is true about urinary incontinence?

    a. It is a normal change of aging.

    b. People experiencing incontinence should limit their fluid intake.

    c. Urinary catheters should be used to manage new onset of incontinence in the hospital.

    d. Constipation can contribute to incontinence.

335. Mrs. Smith, a resident of a local nursing home unit, has lost 10% of her body weight over the past 3 months. Your first intervention should be which of the following?

    a. Do an oral health assessment to determine whether there are oral health problems contributing to her weight loss.

    b. Consult with dietary to order larger portion sizes.

    c. Obtain an order for a dietary supplement.

    d. Notify her physician.

336. Sally Jones has a pressure ulcer that is not healing. You know that which of the following factors can interfere with wound healing?

    a. Nutrition

    b. Cognition

    c. Poor sleep

    d. Excessive movement

337. Which of the following are true statements about normal changes of aging?

    a. All age-related differences result from disease.

    b. When comparing functional abilities of an older adult, it is important not to allow social or cultural factors to cloud your assessment.

    c. It is always very easy to tell the difference between normal changes of aging and the results of poor habits over time.

    d. There can be enormous diversity in every person at every age in every part of the body.

338. When giving care to an older bedridden patient with limited mobility, which intervention is appropriate?

   a. Turn and reposition the patient every 2 hours.

   b. Administer prophylactic antibiotics.

   c. Ensure the placement of multiple IV lines in the event that rapid hydration and blood pressure support becomes necessary.

   d. Draw labs daily to ensure the adequacy of white blood cell response.

339. Mr. Hernandez is an 87-year-old man with a diagnosis of community-acquired pneumonia. His vital signs are 106/78, 82, 24 with an oral temperature of 97 degrees F. His granddaughter asks why he is not running a fever despite the fact that he is so ill. You respond:

   a. "He is no longer febrile because his pneumonia is resolved."

   b. "In older adults 97 degrees F is considered febrile."

   c. "Lack of fever does not mean lack of infection in older adults."

   d. "The oral temperature was probably inaccurate."

340. Presbycusis is defined as:

   a. Thick, dry cerumen

   b. High-pitched ringing in the ears

   c. Loss of ability to hear high-pitched frequencies

   d. Inability to read small print close up

341. Glaucoma is defined as:

   a. A breakdown in the absorption of intraocular fluid leading to an increase in intraocular pressure

   b. A spasm in eye muscles leading to eye pain

   c. A yellowish film over the surface of the lens of the eye

   d. A disorder of the macula that affects central vision

342. What do we know about activity in older adults?

   a. Older adults should limit their activity to avoid injury.

   b. Nonweight-bearing activities can prevent osteoporosis.

   c. Arthritic older adults should avoid physical activity.

   d. None of the above.

343. Causes of sleep problems in older adults can include:

   a. Dementia, depression, and stress

   b. Pain, medications, and urinary incontinence

    c. Medications and chronic illness

    d. All of the above

344. You are a nurse on a medical unit in a large medical center. You use the Fulmer SPICES to assess all of the following *except:*

    a. Sleep

    b. Incontinence

    c. Falls

    d. Social support

345. Which of the following signs would make you suspect a stroke?

    a. Forgetting where the car keys are

    b. Bilateral facial drooping

    c. Unilateral weakness

    d. All of the above

346. In teaching a patient with GERD, which of the following interventions might be used?

    a. Lie down and relax for 30 minutes after eating.

    b. Engage in vigorous exercise after eating.

    c. Consume additional citrus in your diet.

    d. None of the above.

347. You notice the following physiological changes in your newly admitted patient: clubbed fingers, barrel chest, and shortness of breath. You suspect that he may have the following diagnosis:

    a. COPD

    b. Asthma

    c. Pneumonia

    d. Pulmonary emboli

348. Your patient tells you that she does not like to take her eye drops for her glaucoma. She reports that she is having no eye pain. How might you advise her?

    a. "If you start to have pain, you should start to take them again immediately."

    b. "You should not stop taking them because you could lose your vision."

    c. "You can cut back to once per day if you have no pain."

    d. "Eye drops are of little use for your condition."

349. Your mother has been told that she has poor bone density. You anticipate which of the following interventions might be tried *first*?

   a. Dietary changes and weight-bearing exercise

   b. Hormone replacement therapy

   c. An osteoclast inhibitor

   d. A change to a high-protein diet

350. Mrs. Smith is picking up her prescriptions. She has additional insurance to help cover the expense of these prescriptions through:

   a. Medicare A

   b. Medicare B

   c. Medicare C

   d. Medicare D

351. A 92-year-old patient with a diagnosis of advanced Alzheimer's disease is admitted following a fall with a fracture. You are not sure whether she requires pain medication. You should:

   a. Use a validated tool such as the PAINAD.

   b. Ask her to rate her pain on a scale of 0 to 10.

   c. Give her pain medication every 4 hours, to be on the safe side.

   d. Ask her family to rate the level of pain.

352. In order to determine whether a drug is effective, a company has randomly assigned patients to two different groups. One group will get an experimental medication, the other will get a placebo. Outcomes will be measured at the end of the study. This type of study is called:

   a. A randomized controlled trial

   b. A qualitative study

   c. A case study

   d. A quasi-experimental study

353. Mrs. Zipps, a 79-year-old woman, is admitted with unilateral swelling and redness of her right lower calf and is being treated with heparin. You expect that her diagnosis might be:

   a. Congestive heart failure

   b. Deep vein thrombosis

   c. Fracture

   d. Gout

354. Mrs. Johnson has just been admitted following a diagnosis of hip fracture. Which of the following are risk factors for constipation?

   a. Decreased movement

   b. Use of narcotic pain medications

   c. Decreased intake of high-fiber foods

   d. All of the above

355. Which of the following statements about the population of adults older than age 65 is ture?

   a. Most older adults live alone

   b. They comprise the majority of patients on acute care medical–surgical units

   c. More than 10% live in nursing homes

   d. None of the above

356. By the year 2030, approximately what proportion of the U.S. population will be older than age 65?

   a. 1 in 2

   b. 1 in 5

   c. 1 in 10

   d. 1 in 20

357. Which of the following is true about the gender distribution of older adults?

   a. Women have a shorter life span than men.

   b. Men outnumber women.

   c. There are roughly equal numbers of men and women.

   d. Women are more likely to live alone.

358. Which of the following statements is true about cultural diversity among older adults?

   a. Cultural diversity is expected to decline over the next decade.

   b. Cultural diversity will increase over the next decade.

   c. Cultural diversity will remain stable over the next decade.

   d. None of the above.

359. Which states have the highest proportion of older adults?

   a. California, Florida, New Jersey

   b. Florida, Maine, West Virginia

   c. Utah, Colorado, Iowa

   d. New York, New Jersey, Connecticut

360. What effect did the GI Bill have on the current population of older adults?

   a. It increased the number of older adults living in poverty.

   b. In increased the number of men receiving a college education.

   c. It increased the proportion of older adults eligible for coverage by the Department of Veterans Affairs.

   d. None of the above.

361. You are going to see a movie with an older adult at a movie theater. You know which of the following things about her vision:

   a. She will have difficulty seeing the screen due to presbyopia.

   b. She will have difficulty with glare due to arcus senilis.

   c. She will be at an increased risk of falls when moving from bright light into darkness.

   d. She will have difficulty understanding the movie due to normal cognitive changes.

362. You notice that the soup your grandmother made is extremely salty. This could be because:

   a. She is trying to increase her sodium intake to decrease her blood pressure.

   b. She knows that older adults need to be sure to consume enough sodium.

   c. As people age, they can have a decreased perception of salt.

   d. All of the above.

363. What is the number one killer of women older than age 25?

   a. Breast cancer

   b. Coronary artery disease

   c. Cancer

   d. Diabetes

364. Which of the following is a consequence of arteriosclerosis?

    a. Narrowing of arteries causes increased pressure.

    b. Narrowed arteries increase risk of cardiovascular problems.

    c. Increased vascular pressure raises stroke risk.

    d. All of the above.

365. Which of the following nursing interventions would be appropriate for a person with heart failure?

    a. Encourage the patient to consume more salt, since salt can increase cardiac contractility.

    b. Encourage the patient to exercise to the best of his or her ability.

    c. Discourage daily weights, since managing heart failure is more important than monitoring weight.

    d. All of the above.

366. What theory is also known as the biological or genetic clock theory?

    a. Wear and tear

    b. Programmed aging

    c. Cross-linkage

    d. Free radical

367. What theory states that, over time, stressors cause a progressive decline in cellular function and eventually lead to death?

    a. Wear and tear

    b. Programmed aging

    c. Cross-linkage

    d. Immunity

368. Which theory explains why there is a decrease in function of certain cells that, over time, leads to increased rates of infection and cancer with age?

    a. Cross-linkage

    b. Free radical

    c. Immunity

    d. Sociological

369. Which theory explains that, over time, normal metabolic practices lead to the production of charged particles, which can damage cells?

    a. Free radical theory

    b. Cross-linkage

    c. Immunity theory

    d. Wear and tear theory

370. Which theory helps explain why older adults have fewer problems with allergies and graft rejection?

    a. Free radical theory

    b. Cross-linkage

    c. Immunity theory

    d. Wear and tear theory

371. What type of arthritis is characterized by exacerbations and remissions and is associated with severe joint deformities?

    a. Osteoarthritis

    b. Rheumatoid arthritis

    c. Both osteoarthritis and rheumatoid arthritis

    d. Neither osteoarthritis nor rheumatoid arthritis

372. Miguel Hernandez, 79 years old, has been admitted to your nursing home. His medications include Aricept, insulin, atenolol, simvastatin, and Colace. Based solely on this information, you decide to order which type of diet?

    a. A regular diet

    b. A low-fat diet

    c. A low-fat, no-added-sugar diet

    d. A low-fat, no-added-sugar, no-added-salt diet

373. The Beers list is a list of medications that should be avoided in older adults. One reason these medications should be avoided is:

    a. They are not covered by the Medicare Part D drug benefit.

    b. They carry a higher risk of side effects in older adults.

    c. They are more likely to be abused by older adults.

    d. They are more likely to cause allergic reactions in older adults.

374. The caregiver spouse of a patient with Alzheimer's disease mentioned that her spouse wanders at night. Which suggestion might be appropriate?

    a. Advise the caregiver to seek a prescription for a strong sedative to use at night.

    b. Recommend that the patient increase daytime nap time.

    c. Suggest that the caregiver use a restraint at night.

    d. Try increasing daytime activity by taking frequent walks.

375. The scale used to determine the risk of developing a pressure ulcer is called:

    a. The Braden Scale

    b. The Tinetti Scale

    c. The MDS

    d. The Pressure Ulcer Risk Scale (PURS)

376. The Joint Commission is the accrediting body for long-term care facilities. It is responsible for assessing whether an agency provides high-quality care and also monitors which of the following?

    a. Patient dementia and confusion

    b. Quality of nursing research conducted in the agency

    c. Performance and continued improvement in care

    d. Mortality and morbidity statistics

377. A 78-year-old man complains of a gradual inability to hear the television, conversational speech, and high-pitched sounds in both ears. This is a common finding in older adults due to:

    a. Presbycusis

    b. Ménière's disease

    c. Vertigo

    d. Tinnitus

378. The following is considered a normal finding in older adults and may result from increased resistance to ventricular filling during atrial contraction:

    a. S_3

    b. Splitting of diastolic sound

    c. S_4

    d. Atrial gallop

379. Older adults who are long-term care residents often exhibit atypical symptoms of pneumonia, such as:

   a. Chest discomfort, dyspnea, and sore throat

   b. Sore throat, leg discomfort, and fever

   c. Changes in behavior, fatigue, and loss of appetite

   d. Confusion, dyspnea, and tinnitus

380. Your patient, who is 77 years old, has vitamin B_{12} deficiency, rheumatoid arthritis, and hypertension. She has recently been experiencing symptoms of hyperthyroidism, such as:

   a. Tremor, palpitations, and proximal weakness

   b. Decreased appetite, fatigue, and depression

   c. Fatigue, low energy, and sadness

   d. Palpitations, dyspnea, and weight gain

381. Which of the following is an age-related change that occurs in the cardiovascular system?

   a. The mass of the SA node contains only about 30% pacemaker cells.

   b. The blood flow to the coronaries increases.

   c. The heart valves stiffen and become thicker.

   d. Lipofuscin decreases in the aging heart.

382. A 76-year-old patient has a Stage II pressure ulcer on her right buttock. She is incontinent of bowel and bladder. The patient was wearing an adult brief that was soaked in urine and had saturated the dressing to the ulcer. She has had the ulcer for 6 months and it appears to be improving. What are your plans?

   a. Keep the wound clean and covered with a wet to moist dressing, begin a toileting program, and prevent the patient from putting pressure on the wound.

   b. Irrigate the wound with peroxide, rinse with water, pack wound with dressing change every 6 hours, make sure her position changes frequently, catheterize patient with Foley catheter.

   c. Irrigate the wound with peroxide, rinse with water, pack wound with dressing, change every 6 hours, insist on patient being transferred to nursing home, make sure she changes position every hour.

   d. Keep the wound open to air during the day and covered with wet to dry dressing at night, catheterize every 6 hours, make sure she changes position every hour.

383. Which type of nursing theory is abstract and used to connect the four main concepts of nursing?

    a. Nursing grand theory

    b. Nursing conceptual model

    c. Nursing middle range theory

    d. Nursing design theory

384. Dimensions of end-of-life care include:

    a. Physical

    b. Spiritual

    c. Psychological

    d. All of the above

385. You are providing a teaching program on dementia to a group of older adults at a senior center. One of the residents says that her mother had dementia and asks you if she is at higher risk. Your response to her would be:

    a. "No, there is no relationship between family history and dementia."

    b. "No, trisomy 21 is the only proven risk factor for developing dementia."

    c. "Yes, there is a relationship between family history and dementia."

    d. "Yes, but the herpes virus and viral encephalitis are greater risk factors."

386. A type of health care insurance available for purchase by older adults to help pay for health care needs not paid for by Medicare is:

    a. Medicare

    b. Medicaid

    c. Private insurance

    d. Medigap

387. The rate of absorption of drugs in the elderly may be slowed due to:

    a. Decreased peristalsis

    b. Dehydration

    c. Delayed gastric emptying

    d. Increased gastric acidity

388. A 78-year-old man has a bladder scan, which finds a residual of 60 mL after urinating. The average postvoid residual urine increases for older adults and falls between:

   a. 25 and 50 mL

   b. 75 and 100 mL

   c. 10 and 25 mL

   d. 50 and 100 mL

389. An 81-year-old woman complains of dizziness, nausea, presyncope, and problems with balance. After being worked up for the dizziness, the diagnosis given is:

   a. Ménière's disease

   b. Seizure disorder

   c. Benign paroxysmal positional vertigo

   d. Cluster headache

390. An 81-year-old woman is complaining of ulcerations in her mouth that are affecting her eating habits and causing severe pain. As the nurse manager of the unit, you are not surprised to see that she is on which of the following medications?

   a. Rosiglitazone (Avandia)

   b. Prednisone

   c. Alendronate (Fosamax)

   d. Furosemide (Lasix)

391. The role of the nurse manager includes which of the following?

   a. Carrying out the nursing process with each patient who has more than two comorbidities

   b. Following the organization's policies and procedures to generate high-quality care

   c. Meeting with the risk manager to determine the best possible insurance coverage for patients with disability

   d. Procuring funds from philanthropists for the unit's operating budget

392. Patient-centered care is described as part of the mission of most long-term care facilities. What are some characteristics of being patient centered?

   a. Nurse-driven, task-oriented, and cost-effective

   b. Knowledge shared with patient, anticipated patient needs, and customized care

c. Centralized, standardized, and specialty focused

d. Time and task oriented and specialty focused

393. A 67-year-old woman comes to the nursing home's wellness clinic with a blood pressure of 155/98, abdominal obesity, total cholesterol of 266, and a fasting blood sugar of 130. After measuring her weight and height, you are not surprised to determine her body mass index to be 33. She most likely will be diagnosed with:

a. Cushing's syndrome

b. Morbid obesity

c. Metabolic syndrome

d. Syndrome XI

394. The inflicting of pain or injury among older adults is classified as which type of elder mistreatment?

a. Physical

b. Psychological

c. Active neglect

d. Passive neglect

395. Regarding stress incontinence, nurses should know that this type of incontinence:

a. Can be caused by bladder muscle weakness

b. Is also called neurogenic bladder

c. Is a leakage of urine resulting from weakened deltoid muscles

d. Results in the total uncontrolled and continuous loss of urine

396. The geriatric nurse caring for a patient at the end of life knows that:

a. Most older adult patients have resolved all their psychological issues by the time death approaches.

b. Most older adult patients have accomplished all developmental tasks of aging by the time death approaches.

c. End-of-life care often provides an opportunity to help patients complete important psychological and developmental tasks of aging.

d. Discussing unresolved psychological and developmental issues is not appropriate in the nurse–patient relationship.

397. Sleep apnea is frequently seen in geriatric clients and is correlated with other chronic illnesses. Risk factors for sleep apnea include which of the following?

    a. Male gender, COPD, older than 75 years

    b. Male gender, obesity, older than 65 years

    c. Female gender, diabetes mellitus, obesity

    d. Female gender, emphysema, heart failure

398. Many older adults experience constipation due to medications and inactivity. Suggestions for promoting improved bowel health include:

    a. Frequent enemas, suppositories, and Fleets

    b. Exercise routines, liquid protein diets

    c. High fiber in diet, increase fluid intake, exercise routines

    d. Fluid restriction, low fiber in diet

399. Mrs. George is an 84-year-old woman newly admitted to your adult day care center with a low score on the Mini-Mental State Examination. Your first line of treatment for her would be to:

    a. Refer her for comprehensive geriatric services.

    b. Rule out delirium and depression as contributors to altered cognitive function.

    c. Do nothing, because cognitive dysfunction is a normal change of aging.

    d. Recommend the physician administer Aricept.

400. The number of annual elder-abuse cases is estimated to exceed:

    a. 200,000

    b. 500,000

    c. 1,000,000

    d. 10,000,000

401. Immobility and having a prothrombotic condition secondary to cardiovascular disease make older adults vulnerable to developing:

    a. Pulmonary fibrosis

    b. Deep vein thrombosis

    c. Lupus erythematosus

    d. Raynaud's disease

402. An 82-year-old man presents with loss of night vision to the point that he feels he should no longer drive at night. He says "everything seems fuzzy." He most likely will be diagnosed with:

    a. Glaucoma

    b. Macular degeneration

    c. Astigmatism

    d. Cataract

403. One of the main reasons older adults experience adverse drug effects is:

    a. Polypharmacy

    b. Increased hydration level

    c. Decreased fat tissue

    d. Decreased lean body mass

404. Observation of posture is a key component of which of the following body system examination?

    a. Skin

    b. Cardiovascular

    c. Abdominal

    d. Respiratory

405. Older adults with long-term hypothyroidism taking levothyroxine (Synthroid) without regular monitoring are at increased risk for developing:

    a. Coagulopathies

    b. Bradycardia

    c. Hearing loss

    d. Osteoporosis

406. Which of the following testing instruments is used to evaluate orientation, recall, and calculation?

    a. Beck Depression Inventory

    b. Barthel Functional Index

    c. PULSES Profile

    d. Folstein Mini-Mental State Examination

407. One of the residents of an assisted living facility is inquiring how to submit a complaint regarding the living arrangements. Who would be best for this resident to contact?

    a. Ombudsman

    b. Staff nurse

    c. Facility administrator

    d. Manager of grounds keeping

408. Coupled with decreased liver and kidney function, older adults also experience which of the following related to their adrenal gland function?

    a. Increased release of mineralocorticoid response

    b. Increased metabolic clearance of cortisol

    c. Decreased metabolic clearance of cortisol

    d. Increased functioning of the adrenal cortex

409. The withholding of necessities among older adults is classified as which type of elder mistreatment?

    a. Physical

    b. Psychological

    c. Active neglect

    d. Passive neglect

410. The end of life is often associated with which of the following physical symptoms among older adults?

    a. Anxiety

    b. Agitation

    c. Depression

    d. Pain

411. An 87-year-old patient in a long-term care facility has just received his first influenza vaccine. He experiences a moderate hypersensitivity response but does fine with an antihistamine. His daughter explains that he has multiple food allergies. He was most likely allergic to which of the following in the influenza vaccine?

    a. Preservative

    b. Egg albumin

    c. Legume extract

    d. Peanut oil

412. An 83-year-old woman has enjoyed summering at the beach her entire life. She has noticed several hyperpigmented macular lesions over the past 10 years but is most concerned when she notes a rough papular area on her right wrist. This papule is most likely:

   a. Lentigine
   b. Seborrheic keratosis
   c. Actinic keratosis
   d. Acrochordons

413. Nurses at a long-term care facility requested professional development on leadership. The nurse manager should do which of the following to fulfill this need?

   a. Teach the nurses about the leadership skills that will help them become nurse managers.
   b. Have the administrator of the facility teach the nurses what she learned in her business program.
   c. Perform a needs survey of the staff to determine what they want to gain regarding leadership skills.
   d. Tell the staff they do not need leadership development unless they want to be a nurse manager.

414. Which of the following is the *most* important use of the information obtained from the functional assessment?

   a. Providing data to develop a medication administration record
   b. Identifying specific self-care deficits
   c. Classifying patient anxiety levels
   d. Determining the cause of the disease process

415. Older adults with type 2 diabetes mellitus who have renal insufficiency should not be prescribed:

   a. Pioglitazone (Actos)
   b. Rosiglitazone (Avandia)
   c. Metformin (Glucophage)
   d. Insulin (Lantus)

416. With older adults, many drugs' half-lives are increased due to:

   a. Coagulopathy
   b. Decreased liver function
   c. Increased liver function
   d. Increased total body water

417. A 71-year-old woman has just had her annual gynecological exam and is surprised to find out that she has bacterial vaginosis. She is sexually active with her husband and says she has noticed a slight odor but did not realize it was abnormal. She has recently finished an antibiotic for an upper respiratory infection. She is more susceptible to this infection due to:

    a. An active sex life

    b. Increased estrogen levels

    c. Changes in the vaginal flora

    d. Atrophy of the vaginal epithelium

418. It is important to assess older adults taking diuretics for symptoms of urinary incontinence, such as:

    a. Dysuria, nocturia, and anuria

    b. Anuria, malodorous urine, and cloudy urine

    c. Urinary frequency, urgency, and nocturia

    d. Dysuria, polyuria, and cloudy urine

419. Older adults normally have a PaO_2 lower than younger adults. The normal range of oxygen for older adults is:

    a. 80 to 89 mmHg

    b. 70 to 75 mmHg

    c. 85 to 90 mmHg

    d. 90 to 95 mmHg

420. An effective means of nutritional assessment is:

    a. 24-hour recall

    b. Forced hydration

    c. Food guide pyramid

    d. Tube feedings

421. Delirium:

    a. Is reversible

    b. Is irreversible

    c. Is part of the normal aging process

    d. Develops over a long period of time

422. Many unsuccessful nurse managers have authority as identified in their job description. They are unable to lead their units successfully if their authority is not linked with which of the following characteristics?

    a. Power

    b. Common sense

    c. Time-management ability

    d. Organizational skills

423. More than one half of all people older than 65 years have cataracts. What are their most common complaints?

    a. Strabismus and diplopia

    b. Diminished visual acuity and glare

    c. Diplopia and loss of color perception

    d. Blindness and floaters

424. Inflammation of the gums and oral soft tissue due to buildup of bacterial plaque causes:

    a. Stomatitis

    b. Aphthous ulceration

    c. Gingivitis

    d. Achalasia

425. An 88-year-old patient often complains of leg cramping that is very painful when he walks but says he has no pain in his legs at rest. He is most likely experiencing:

    a. Venous insufficiency

    b. Restless legs syndrome

    c. Intermittent claudication

    d. Deep vein thrombosis

426. Inflicting mental anguish among older adults is classified as which type of elder mistreatment?

    a. Physical

    b. Psychological

    c. Active neglect

    d. Passive neglect

427. A 78-year-old man is admitted to a long-term care residence with Alzheimer's disease. He is in the final stages of the disease and exhibits which of the following symptoms?

   a. Short-term memory loss, headaches, hearing loss

   b. Memory loss, mood changes, weight loss

   c. Headaches, long-term memory loss, incontinence

   d. Memory loss, vision loss, behavior changes

428. Which dimension of care is most often ignored in end-of-life care plans for older adults?

   a. Physical

   b. Spiritual

   c. Psychological

   d. Social

429. It is significant to observe all patients who have diabetes for signs and symptoms of hypoglycemia, especially when they may have the flu or are dehydrated. These signs and symptoms include:

   a. Confusion, tremors, weakness, diaphoresis

   b. Irritability, hunger, thirst, hearing dysfunction

   c. Diaphoresis, thirst, seizures, behavioral changes

   d. Dementia, rash, chest discomfort, headache

430. When assessing an older adult's ability to function with activities of daily living, it is essential that the interviewer be consistent in assessing for:

   a. Either performance or capacity

   b. The best possible performance of the individual

   c. The individual's ability to function without medications

   d. The individual's ability to function without assistive devices

431. In discussing a functional assessment during a team conference, which of the following statements would the nurse most likely make?

   a. "A functional assessment is used to evaluate the overall ability of older adults to independently complete their activities of daily living."

   b. "The major emphasis of a functional assessment is on psychosocial well-being."

c. "A functional assessment is not necessary until the older adult becomes familiar with the environment."

d. "Many times, the functional assessment can be delegated to a nursing assistant."

432. The most common type of bone fracture with the highest rate of complications in older adults is:

a. Wrist

b. Femur

c. Humerus

d. Hip

433. Which of the following theorists focused on caring as the central essence of nursing?

a. Brenner and Wrubel

b. Hildegard Peplau

c. Madeleine Leininger

d. Martha Rogers

434. A 77-year-old nursing home resident is complaining of a tingling and very painful rash on the left side only in the mid-scapular area of his back. He is diagnosed with herpes zoster and is put on an antiviral drug. He still complains of the pain so you notify the physician, who prescribes which of the following?

a. Acetaminophen (Tylenol)

b. Amitriptyline (Elavil)

c. Prednisone

d. Fexofenadine (Allegra)

435. You have been asked to give a health-teaching program on best dietary practices with iron-deficiency anemia. You will discuss which appropriate foods?

a. Bananas

b. Eggs

c. Legumes and dried fruit

d. Dried pasta

436. Which statement most adequately describes the spiritual needs of older adults at the end of life?

    a. Spirituality may provide a framework within which older adults search for meaning and purpose in life.

    b. Symptom management at the end of life is more important than attention to spiritual needs.

    c. Accomplishing developmental and psychological tasks at the end of life is more important than accomplishing spiritual tasks.

    d. Spiritual care is only important for patients who are deeply religious.

437. Which of the following is a normal, age-related change related to the nervous system?

    a. An increase in the number of functional neurons

    b. A steady loss of intellectual functioning

    c. A gradual decline of sensory perception

    d. An increase in nerve conduction fibers, causing greater sensitivity to pain

438. A 66-year-old man complains of fatigue, malaise, headaches, and an anterior neck mass. He is diagnosed with Hodgkin's lymphoma after many tests. One diagnostic finding in the cells of Hodgkin's lymphoma is:

    a. Philadelphia factor

    b. Cytokine-A

    c. Interferon B

    d. Reed-Sternberg cells

439. Older adults experiencing abdominal discomfort and altered bowel habits are generally diagnosed with which of the following conditions after normal gastrointestinal diagnostic testing?

    a. Crohn's disease

    b. Ulcerative colitis

    c. Spastic colon

    d. Irritable bowel disease

440. The most common outcome of poor compliance among older adults not following their medication regimen is:

    a. Overdosing

    b. Underdosing

    c. Family members using older adult's prescriptions

    d. Toxicity

441. You are bathing an 80-year-old man and you notice that his skin is thin and has reduced elasticity. This finding is related to which normal change of aging?

    a. Integumentary system changes

    b. Increases in elastin and subcutaneous fat

    c. An increase in the number of sweat and sebaceous glands

    d. Increased vascular flow to the skin

442. Older adults in respiratory failure often have a shallow and rapid breathing pattern or a slower respiratory rate. This further increases potential complications because of:

    a. Insufficient CO_2 removal

    b. Compensatory respiratory alkalosis

    c. Decreased lung recoil

    d. Increased vital capacity

443. Older patients on digoxin are most likely to experience the following side effect:

    a. Jaundice

    b. Tinnitus

    c. Confusion

    d. Weight gain

444. Loss of central vision due to macular degeneration is thought to be caused by trauma, aging, and infection. Symptoms of this eye problem include:

    a. Diminished central vision (scotoma), distorted images

    b. Decreased peripheral vision, diplopia, floaters

    c. Poor night vision, distorted images, loss of peripheral vision

    d. Astigmatism, myopia, distorted images

445. Older adults taking opiate narcotics need to be carefully assessed for:

    a. Diarrhea

    b. Constipation

    c. Abdominal cramping

    d. Flatus

446. Many older adults in long-term care facilities experience UTIs. Which organism is most often the pathology?

    a. *Staphylococcus saprophyticus*

    b. *Streptococcus pneumoniae*

    c. *Escherichia coli*

    d. *Enterobacter*

447. Eye examinations for older adults should be referred to ophthalmologists and optometrists if which of the following is suspected?

    a. Cataracts and macular degeneration

    b. Glaucoma and risk of falling

    c. Glaucoma and vertigo

    d. Cerumen impaction and cataracts

448. All nurses have the potential to develop leadership skills. Some examples of leadership skills include:

    a. Managing the budget, orientation of new staff, and establishing safety policies

    b. Motivating staff, empowering others to lead, and creating a vision

    c. Motivating others, assisting all staff to be educated, and managing the schedule

    d. Registering all staff for educational programs, recommending staff become certified, and creating a strategic plan for the organization

449. Medicare and Medicaid legislation are examples of which of the following periods in U.S. health care history?

    a. 1940 to 1950

    b. 1960 to 1970

    c. 1980 to 1990

    d. 1990 to 2000

450. A key finding of the Institute of Medicine report, *The Future of Nursing* is that:

    a. The terminal degree of the nursing profession should be the PhD.

    b. Nurses involved in independent practice should avoid collaborations with nonnurse providers of care, such as nurse-extenders.

    c. The LPN/LVN is the educational standard for the hospital staff nurse.

    d. Nurses should practice to the fullest extent of their education and training.

451. In your discharge teaching for a patient with heart failure you use concepts from activity theory in providing discharge education when you suggest that the patient should:

    a. Continue a daily walking routine

    b. Be sure to confine herself to bed rest until she is feeling better

    c. Limit contact with crowds and young children

    d. Get a flu shot

452. A 73-year-old woman is found to have a hemoglobin A1C level of 8.5. You know that this is indicative of:

    a. Excellent glycemic control

    b. Poor glycemic control

    c. A1C is not able to provide information about glycemic control over time

    d. Excellent compliance with diet, exercise, and medication recommendations

453. Which of the following is a common cause of delirium?

    a. Anesthetic medication

    b. Urinary retention

    c. Quiet surroundings

    d. Genetics

454. Which of the following are valid ways to assess pain in a cognitively intact patient?

    a. Ask the patient to rate the pain on a pain scale.

    b. Ask the patient to rate the pain on a pain scale, knowing that patients commonly overestimate their pain.

    c. Use both a pain scale combined with your nursing judgment about what an appropriate level of pain should be for a given disease or condition in order to determine the patient's actual level of pain.

    d. All of the above

455. Signs and symptoms of malnutrition in older adults can include:

    a. Decreased weight

    b. Increased number of wounds

    c. Increased serum albumin

    d. Both a and b

456. Which of the following medications is associated with delirium in older adults?

   a. Hydromorphone and diphenhydramine

   b. Atenolol and metoprolol

   c. Docusate sodium

   d. All of the above

457. When a nurse tells the truth about a patient's terminal condition she is engaging in

   a. Beneficence

   b. Autonomy

   c. Veracity

   d. Fidelity

458. A nurse is assigned to care for a patient who is terminally ill with COPD. The respirations of the patient have slowed and the patient is severely anxious, in pain, and short of breath. The nurse is concerned about medicating the patient for pain because she knows that giving the pain medication to treat the patient's symptoms may, in fact, hasten the death of the patient. Which of the following can help inform her decision?

   a. It is legal and ethical to give a medication to treat symptoms at the end of life, even if giving that medication may hasten death.

   b. If a medication is given that hastens death, it is considered euthanasia and is illegal.

   c. The nurse must consider the legal consequences of her actions, as giving the medication is not legal.

   d. Although legal, the nurse may still lose her license for giving the medication as it is a clear violation of the ANA *Code of Ethics*.

459. Which of the following communication strategies is appropriate for a patient with presbycusis?

   a. Use a slightly lower tone of voice, repeat information as necessary.

   b. Pose all questions to the patient's spouse.

   c. Avoid verbal communication, instead rely on nonverbal cues.

   d. All of the above

460. First-generation psychiatric or neuroleptic medications are more likely to be associated with which side effect?

a. Pain

b. UTIs

c. Tardive dyskinesia

d. Diaphoresis

461. You are about to discharge your patient to her home. She will need to be able to change the dressing on an abdominal wound daily. Effective teaching of this patient would include:

a. Having the patient explain the dressing change procedure

b. Having the patient return demonstrate the dressing change

c. Providing the patient with written instructions about the dressing change

d. All of the above

462. Alzheimer's disease is more common in:

a. People with a genetic predisposition

b. Patients with Down syndrome

c. Patients older than age 80

d. All of the above

463. Which of the following behaviors demonstrates that a nurse values patient autonomy?

a. Allowing a resident to choose what to eat for lunch

b. Selecting lunch items for the resident that will allow the patient to lose weight

c. Ensuring that the patient will have the opportunity to eat after you have finished providing nursing care

d. None of the above

464. A 76-year-old overweight male complains of osteoarthritis in the left knee. The patient is referred for a nutritional consultation because:

a. Weight loss can help improve symptoms of osteoarthritis.

b. Obesity is an absolute contraindication to joint replacement.

c. Certain foods may aggravate osteoarthritis.

d. Obesity creates intolerance to pain medication.

465. The major difference between a TIA and a CVA is that:
    a. TIA symptoms resolve more quickly.
    b. TIA symptoms always precede a CVA.
    c. TIA symptoms do not usually involve facial drooping.
    d. CVA symptoms resolve more quickly.

466. Allowing a patient to decide when to get up in the morning demonstrates a commitment to:
    a. Autonomy
    b. Justice
    c. Fidelity
    d. Veracity

467. HIPAA rules are concerned with:
    a. Autonomy
    b. Fidelity
    c. Veracity
    d. Confidentiality

468. A common reason a nursing home patient might be deficient in vitamin D might be:
    a. Lack of sun exposure
    b. Lactose intolerance
    c. Feeling cold and covering up when outdoors
    d. All of the above

469. Mrs. Johnson, a 94-year-old woman with a diagnosis of moderate to severe Alzheimer's disease, has been losing weight at the nursing home. Which of the following interventions should be tried first?
    a. Contact her prescriber for an order for a nutritional supplement, such as Ensure.
    b. Increase the level of feeding assistance provided.
    c. Change her to a high-fat, high-calorie diet.
    d. Decrease the number of snacks throughout the day, so that she will be more hungry at mealtime.

470. Physical changes in the older women that affect sexual activity include:

    a. Enlargement of the breast

    b. Decreased lubrication of the vaginal mucosa

    c. Increase in the production of estrogen

    d. Impotence

471. Which of the following is true about medications used to treat Alzheimer's disease?

    a. They have very few side effects.

    b. They are highly effective in the treatment of advanced dementia.

    c. The most common side effect is gastrointestinal disturbance.

    d. They carry a high risk of stroke.

472. How might you begin a conversation with an older adult about sexual health?

    a. "Would it be okay for me to ask you some questions about your sexual health?"

    b. "Tell me your concerns about fulfilling your continuing sexual needs."

    c. "I assume that you don't have any questions, but if you do, let me know."

    d. "Most older adults are not sexually active, but let me know if you are."

473. The physician has ordered Coumadin for your poststroke patient. What does this tell you?

    a. The patient arrived in the ER less than 6 hours following the onset of symptoms.

    b. The patient had a hemorrhagic stroke that can be helped by medication.

    c. The patient is likely also suffering from a myocardial infarction.

    d. The patient had a stroke caused by a thrombus.

474. Restraints may be in all of the following forms, *except*:

    a. Bed alarms

    b. Lap buddies

    c. Mittens

    d. IV boards

475. In discussing age-related changes associated with excretion, the nurse knows that:

   a. Age does not affect the excretion of drugs to any appreciable degree.

   b. When the kidneys are not functioning properly, drugs tend to remain in the bloodstream longer, increasing the risk of toxicity.

   c. Most drugs are not affected by kidney functioning.

   d. The GFR in the kidney increases with age, resulting in an increase in the excretion of drugs.

476. The nurse must be aware of the following age-related changes that affect continence. With age:

   a. There is an increase in bladder capacity

   b. There is a decrease in bladder muscle tone

   c. There is a decrease in residual volume

   d. There is an increased in the perception of the urge to void

477. Which of the following is true about how Americans die?

   a. Most wish to die at home

   b. About 25% die at home

   c. About 75% die at home

   d. Both a and b

478. Which of the following normal age-related changes increase the risk of pneumonia in an older adult?

   a. Decreased number of cilia

   b. Decreased cough reflex

   c. Increased risk of aspiration

   d. All of the above

479. Normal age-related changes in the integument include:

   a. Increased elasticity

   b. Increased perspiration

   c. Decreased tissue thickness

   d. All of the above

480. Which of the following is an age-related change that occurs within the gastrointestinal system?

   a. Decreased rate of peristalsis
   b. Increased gastric acid production
   c. The gut valves stiffen and become thicker
   d. Lipofuscin decreases in the aging gut

481. Which of the following changes in the skeletal system is least characteristic of normal aging?

   a. Decreased range of motion
   b. Loss of height of up to 10 cm
   c. Chronic inflammation of the joints
   d. Loss of some muscle mass

482. An age-related change of the musculoskeletal system is:

   a. Decrease in height with posture becoming straighter and more defined.
   b. The lengthening of the spinal column resulting in kyphosis.
   c. Muscle fibers shortening and increasing in number.
   d. Bone reabsorption causing the bone to lose calcium causing decreased ability to produce material for the bone matrix.

483. Which of the following statements is true about physical restraints?

   a. Physical restraints help prevent older adults from falling.
   b. A bed alarm is a type of physical restraint.
   c. Confused older adults are more at risk for physical restraints than older adults who are not confused.
   d. Most older adults who have been physically restrained do not suffer any psychological trauma from the treatment.

484. Mrs. Smith has a hematocrit of 65. You realize this is likely:

   a. A gastrointestinal bleed
   b. A normal change of aging
   c. A consequence of hypovolemia
   d. Because of malnutrition

485. Which of the following questions about sleep is most appropriately posed?

a. "Do you have difficulty sleeping?"

b. "You are not having any trouble sleeping, are you?"

c. "Tell me about your sleep."

d. "I notice that sometimes you use sleeping pills at home. Can I order you some while you are here in the hospital?"

486. Which of the following is true about pain at the end of life?

a. At the end of life, most people cannot feel pain.

b. It is both legal and ethical to administer pain medication to a dying patient, even if the final dose of pain medication results in his or her death.

c. Pain at the end of life is generally well managed.

d. None of the above

487. Restraints should rarely (if ever) be used in long-term care facilities. However, which of the following situations is an acceptable reason for using restraints on an older adult?

a. When the patient wants to get out of bed to go to the bathroom several times per night

b. When the patient is restless and has no order for a sedative

c. When the patient is cognitively impaired

d. To ensure the physical safety of the patient or other patients

488. Of the following nursing interventions for fall prevention, which is not helpful?

a. Minimize clutter in the environment

b. Physical restraints

c. Strengthening exercises

d. Walking

489. Mrs. Jones is starting a medication that is negatively affected by eating high amounts of vitamin K. Which foods should she avoid?

a. Oranges

b. Spinach

c. Bananas

d. Oatmeal

490. All of the following increase the risk score on the Braden Scale *except:*

   a. Increased moisture

   b. Poor nutrition

   c. Decreased mobility

   d. Poor staffing

491. Lower levels of RN staffing are associated with which of the following outcomes?

   a. Increased rate of pressure ulcers

   b. Increased rate of antipsychotic use

   c. Higher fall rates

   d. All of the above

492. Which of the following is an example of a modifiable risk factor?

   a. Age

   b. Menopausal status

   c. Obesity

   d. Family history

493. Which of the following patient groups should not receive the shingles vaccine?

   a. People with a weakened immune system

   b. Patients who have already had shingles

   c. Patients older than age 60

   d. A patient who has already had chicken pox

494. A patient who is incontinent because he or she is physically unable to get to the bathroom is said to have:

   a. Stress incontinence

   b. Functional incontinence

   c. Overflow incontinence

   d. Urge incontinence

495. A 75-year-old male with a 25 pack-year smoking history and a diagnosis of COPD is most likely to have which of the following conditions?

   a. Metabolic alkalosis

   b. Metabolic acidosis

   c. Respiratory alkalosis

   d. Respiratory acidosis

496. Which of the following is true about sexuality among older adults?

    a. Older women may experience an absence of older male partners.

    b. Sexual desires diminish with age.

    c. In general, sexual patterns change significantly as people age.

    d. All of the above

497. You have a patient who has rated her pain as 9/10. The patient has MS Contin 15 mg twice a day. The last dose was at 9 a.m. and it is now 2 p.m. The patient is asking for more pain medication. What should you do?

    a. Administer the MS Contin early

    b. Contact the prescriber

    c. Employ nonpharmacologic methods of pain control such as a back rub

    d. Kindly explain to the patient that the next dose of medication will not be due until 9 p.m.

498. You are caring for an older gentleman at the end of life who has been receiving large doses of morphine for several months to control metastatic bone pain. You notice that his respirations have slowed significantly, but he is still moaning in pain. He has an order for MS 10 mg SL as needed every 2 hours. His last dose of MS was 6 hours ago. What do you do?

    a. Administer the Narcan to reverse the effects of the narcotic and improve the respiratory rate

    b. Administer the MS even though you know that it may hasten death

    c. Hold the MS until the respiratory rate improves

    d. Contact the prescriber

499. You are caring for a patient at the end of life who has been receiving MS Contin, 30 mg orally twice a day. You go in to administer his morning dose and your assessment reveals that he is not able to safely swallow his MS Contin. What do you do?

    a. Crush the MS Contin and give it with applesauce

    b. Start an IV and administer the equivalent amount of morphine IV push

    c. Hold the MS Contin until the patient can safely swallow

    d. Contact the prescriber for an order for morphine sulfate SL

500. Diabetics frequently experience neuropathic pain and obtain effective relief from drugs from which of the following categories?

    a. Opiates

    b. Antiepileptics

    c. NSAIDs

Posttest Answers and Rationales

1. **d.** Unequal pupillary constriction in response to light

   Increases in eyebrow hair are seen in men as a result of hormonal shifts. An arcus senilis is caused by a buildup of cholesterol around the iris. It does not affect the vision and is considered a normal change of aging. Decreases in tear production, sweat, and saliva are normal. Pupillary constriction should always be equal in both eyes, therefore it is the only abnormal change.

2. **a.** Graying of America

   Maximum life span is defined as the longest amount of time from birth to death for a given species, whereas life expectancy is the average amount of time a person is expected to live. The correct answer, "a," refers to the fact that the nation as a whole is getting older, hence, "graying."

3. **c.** Manage disease so it does not get worse

   Preventing disease before it occurs is primary prevention. Detecting disease at an earlier stage is secondary prevention. Managing disease so it does not get worse is tertiary prevention.

4. **b.** Increases contractility and decreases heart rate

   One of the primary side effects of a beta blocker is to decrease heart rate. Prior to administering a beta blocker, the nurse should assess heart rate and hold the medication if the heart rate is below 60.

5. **c.** Fever

Cough and pedal edema are classic symptoms of heart failure in an older adult. Confusion may also be present, as the disease can decrease oxygenation to the brain. Fever is not a symptom of heart failure in older adults.

6. **c.** Motivational theory

The Herzberg theory states that certain factors may not increase motivation (e.g., comfortable chairs). However, if these factors are absent motivation can decrease.

7. **a.** Increased excretion through the urinary tract

As people age, their GFR decreases. Therefore, medications will tend to be retained, not excreted. The other answers—decreased absorption, decreased metabolism, and decreased renal clearance—are all important considerations when administering medications to older adults.

8. **c.** Gout

Allopurinol (Zyloprim) and bethanechol (Urecholine) are medications specifically used in the treatment of gout. Gout is a genetically based disorder, more common in men, which results in the inability to break down purines.

9. **c.** Mission, philosophy, and goals of the organization

An understanding of the mission, philosophy and goals of the organization is an important accreditation standard. Although each of the other answer choices may or may not be discussed, they are not mandated.

10. **b.** Septic arthritis secondary to gonorrhea and chlamydia

The patient's sexual history should lead you to think about sexually transmitted diseases. Osteopenia and osteoporosis do not result in fever. Sarcoidosis, an inflammatory condition found typically in the lungs or lymph nodes, does not fit this symptom profile. Osteomyelitis, a bone infection, would present with a different symptom profile.

11. **c.** Cough

It is important to know that in older adults, conditions may often present in an atypical manner. Cough, a cardinal sign of pneumonia in younger people, may be absent in older adults.

12. **c.** Transactional

Transactional leadership is a style that encourages compliance through rewards and punishments. It is an authoritative style of leadership. Both democratic and transformational leadership put more weight on the value of individual opinions and preferences to implement systematic changes. Laissez-faire leadership is a style of "hands off" leadership.

13. **d.** Capsaicin cream

   Capsaicin cream is the only drug approved for the treatment of postherpetic neuralgia. Meperidine (Demerol) is a medication from the Beers list that should not be used in older adults, and is largely considered ineffective for this condition. Acyclovir (Zovirax) is an antiviral drug used in the initial phase of the condition, and is recommended during the first 72 hours. It is not an effective long-term treatment.

14. **c.** Cellulitis

   The key symptoms, the presence of swelling and erythematous streaks, indicate cellulitis.

15. **d.** Selected so that each member of a population has an equal probability of being included

   A random sample is one in which every member of a given population has an equal probably of being selected into a sample. The sample would only be representative of the average American, if every American had an equal probably of being selected. This is, in fact, unlikely. A sample chosen on the basis of convenience is called a convenience sample.

16. **a.** Adherence

   Adherence or compliance describes the degree to which a patient follows a given treatment plan. Health literacy can affect the degree of adherence to a protocol.

17. **c.** The older adult

   The primary source of information about patients should be the patients themselves. An older adult's self-report should be considered the gold standard provided that there is no evidence of cognitive impairment.

18. **d.** To ensure the physical safety of the patient or other patients

   The only viable answer is "d". It is important that restraints never be used for any of the other reasons. If restraints need to be used to ensure safety, they should only be employed temporarily, until other, better methods can be used.

19. **c.** Between 3 to 6 months posttransplant

   The most common time to develop graft versus host disease is 3 to 6 months following treatment.

20. **c.** Keep a daily written log of exercise and include type of exercise, time of exercise, and the intensity of exercise

   Keeping an exercise log will help a patient track his or her exercise, set goals, and monitor progress. The other answer choices are contraindicated and are dangerous.

21. **d.** Institutional review board

   Institutional review board approval is required prior to beginning any research study.

22. **b.** Vitamin B_{12}

   Vitamin B_{12} deficiency can cause anemia, fatigue, memory, and neurological problems. It can be caused by lack of intake or the lack of ability to absorb B_{12}.

23. **b.** Medicare

   Because the patient is older than 65 and in the hospital, Medicare is the primary insurer.

24. **a.** Anxiety

   Although the other symptoms may be present at the end of life, anxiety is the only *psychological* symptom.

25. **a.** Protection from injury

   A priority intervention for all patients is safety. Thus, protection from injury is the correct answer.

26. **d.** Protect patient privacy

   HIPAA regulations are intended to prevent disclosure of patient information to individuals who are not directly involved with the care of a patient.

27. **a.** Successful aging is an extension of an individual's developmental patterns throughout life

   Continuity theory suggests that older adults tend to maintain the same coping strategies that they did when they were younger. Therefore, successful aging rests on the development of these core coping strategies.

28. **a.** Application of heat and/or cold—whichever is effective

   Both heat and cold can be effective in the management of osteoarthritis. NSAIDs can be taken with food every 6 hours, however, they may increase the risk of bleeding and stroke.

29. b. Complications leading to death

Older adults with pneumonia are at higher risk of complications than are younger adults. They are less likely to develop fever than younger adults.

30. d. Disorientation

One of the key characteristics separating the diagnosis of delirium from dementia is onset. Dementia demonstrates a gradual onset, whereas delirium is a disorientation that occurs acutely.

31. d. Kaposi's sarcoma

Although HIV-positive patients are more susceptible to infectious skin diseases, the purple colored popular rash is indicative of Kaposi's sarcoma.

32. b. ACE inhibitor

ACE inhibitors are first-line therapy for patients with heart failure.

33. c. Decreased GFR

GFR decreases with age.

34. a. Prevent disease before it occurs

The purpose of primary prevention is to prevent disease before it occurs. Secondary prevention provides optimal management of disease, so that it does not progress. Tertiary prevention focuses on mitigating negative consequences of disease.

35. c. Osteoarthritis and osteoporosis

Osteoarthritis and osteoporosis are two of the most common skeletal diseases of aging.

36. d. All of the above

Nurses should understand that there are many reasons why a patient may not report pain. Therefore, careful assessment and thoughtful communication about pain are critical.

37. a. Periodontal disease

Although periodontal disease is not a normal part of aging, it is associated with other dental problems. A decrease in the production of saliva (not mucus) is considered to be a normal change of aging.

38. d. Encourage religious and spiritual practices at the end of life

Nurses should ensure that older adults have the means to engage in spiritual practices to the extent possible. This is important throughout the aging process, however, it is particularly important at the end of life.

39. c. Evidence-based practice

Nurses should be able to read and apply research to address clinical problems.

40. d. Dizziness and tinnitus

Dizziness and tinnitus are associated with Ménière's disease.

41. b. Increase the brain's level of acetylcholine

Cholinesterase inhibitors decrease the function of the enzyme cholinesterase (which serves the primary function of breaking down acetylcholine). By inhibiting cholinesterase, more acetylcholine can accumulate in the synaptic cleft, thereby increasing neurological function.

42. a. Line of authority from the administrator to the unlicensed assistive personnel

The organizational structure should *not* be simply reflective of the nursing personnel, but reflect all members of the organization from the administrator to the unlicensed assistive personnel (and everyone in between).

43. c. Area Agencies on Aging

The Area Agencies on Aging were formed by Title III of the older Americans Act. Medicare, Title XVIII, was established as part of the Social Security Act. Medicaid, Title XIX, was added to the Social Security Act.

44. c. NSAIDs

NSAIDs are associated with a high risk of gastrointestinal bleeding. They should be taken together with food.

45. b. Is blunted with age

The febrile response in older adults is blunted with age. This is because of both a diminished white blood cell response and a diminished hypothalamic response to generate a fever.

46. c. Heberden's nodes

Heberden's nodes are enlarged joints that occur at the end of the fingers. The presence of Heberden's nodes, therefore, can impact fine motor skills.

47. b. AARP

With more than 30 million members, AARP is the nation's largest and most powerful advocacy group.

48. a. Are nursing actions that will assist the patient to meet the identified goals

Nursing interventions should be tied to the nursing diagnosis and performed with the objective of meeting a patient goal.

49. c. Beers Criteria

The Beers Criteria provide a list of medications that are potentially unsafe in older adults.

50. c. Decreased bladder capacity

Decreased mobility and decreased cognition can impact continence in older adults, but they are not considered normal changes of aging. Decreased bladder capacity, when combined with other factors, can be a contributing factor for incontinence.

51. b. "I am just too tired to do anything."

Depression in older adults can sometimes be masked in the context of other comorbid conditions. If an older adult discloses that he or she is feeling too tired to do anything, or is feeling unmotivated to do the things that once brought him or her pleasure, a follow-up screening, such as the Geriatric Depression Scale (GDS), should be performed.

52. b. LDL should be less than 100

LDL is considered "bad" cholesterol. It should be less than 100. HDL or "good" cholesterol should be greater than 50. Triglyceride levels should be less than 150.

53. c. Bathing

Any actions that require nursing judgment cannot be delegated. Therefore, the only possible answer is bathing.

54. b. Detect disease at an earlier, more treatable stage

Secondary prevention consists of early diagnosis together with rapid and effective treatment.

55. b. Healthy People 2020

Healthy People 2020 is the name of the guideline with set goals for the health of the nation. There was a previous iteration of this initiative known as Healthy People 2010.

56. c. Kegel exercises

Kegel exercises are intended to strengthen the pelvic floor; therefore, they can be a useful intervention for stress incontinence.

57. **b.** Names a person for making health care decisions on behalf of the patient

   A durable power of attorney names a person to make health care decisions should a patient be unable to do so. A living will, on the other hand, spells out a patient's desires for life-sustaining treatment.

58. **d.** Decreased vascular compliance

   As a person ages, the arteries can harden and become more rigid. This, combined with decreased baroreceptor functionality, can result in increases in blood pressure.

59. **c.** Prednisone

   Temporal arteritis, also called giant cell arteritis, is an inflammatory condition of the blood vessels feeding the temporal area of the head. It is treated with anti-inflammatory medications to prevent vascular occlusion.

60. **d.** Rosacea

   Given the patient's age and history, rosacea should be considered.

61. **a.** Fewer killer T cells in the immunologic system

   Older adults produce fewer "killer" T cells in response to infection than younger people do. This change can also decrease responsiveness to vaccines, and increase the risk of a variety of other infections.

62. **a.** Increased cost of medication

   Older adults are likely to take multiple medications to manage chronic conditions. Approximately 29% of older adults take five or more medications daily.

63. **a.** Carbohydrates

   Although older adults with type 2 diabetes should have a good understanding of nutrition, including fats, it is carbohydrate intake that will most directly affect postprandial glucose levels.

64. **a.** The "wear and tear" theory

   "Wear and tear" theory is the only *biological* theory listed. Test takers would be well advised to have an understanding of the different theories mentioned in Chapter 3.

65. **b.** Lack of energy, fatigue, and malaise

   Lack of energy, fatigue, and malaise are common symptoms experienced after infection. Older adults tend not to manifest fever, and chest discomfort together with fatigue are characteristic of other cardiac problems.

66. **d.** Iron

    Decreases in iron absorption can lead to microcytic, hypochromic anemia in older adults.

67. **b.** Sign up for exercise class, get some sun, and do yoga

    Research has suggested that exercise and sunlight have powerful effects on mood. A social exercise class, like yoga, can also help establish critical social connections.

68. **b.** "If there is no vitamin K in it, you can take it."

    Although it is usually not necessary for older adults to take supplementary vitamins, as long as the multivitamin does not contain vitamin K, it should be safe to take together with Coumadin.

69. **c.** An elderly person may not exhibit outward signs of pain even when he or she is actually experiencing pain

    Older adults often do not exhibit outward signs of pain, and may be less likely to report pain when it is present. Pain is not a normal consequence of aging. On a pain scale, 0 represents no pain and 10 represents the worst possible pain.

70. **c.** Malignancies and tuberculosis

    Anemia of chronic disease occurs as the result of a struggle of the immune system to fight off disease, malignancy, or as in the case of autoimmune diseases, to fight the host body itself. Anemia of chronic disease is different than the anemia that results from renal failure.

71. **b.** OASIS assessment

    In home care the assessment done for patients is called the OASIS assessment. In nursing homes, the resident assessment is called the MDS.

72. **d.** All of the above

    There can be many reasons an older adult may withhold information during an assessment. Providers should communicate that they are interested in all facets of the patient's history.

73. **a.** Actinic keratosis

    These keratose are found on areas exposed to sunlight, such as the face and hands. Although they are not cancerous, they may develop into malignancies over time.

74. **d.** Keep up the good work!

    A high HDL is a good sign, and is considered to be cardio-protective.

75. **b.** Adverse effects of polypharmacy

   Polypharmacy is a common problem for older adults. In addition, older adults are at risk of problems with falls, hydration, and poor hearing. We tend not to focus on the body-image issues of older adults in nursing homes.

76. **d.** Loss of elasticity of the lens

   Presbyopia refers to a difficulty in viewing near objects. It is caused by a loss of elasticity of the lens. Although the reaction time of the pupil does decline, this causes difficulty in accommodating rapid changes in light and dark.

77. **d.** Gastrointestinal

   NSAIDs should be taken with food to avoid gastrointestinal distress.

78. **c.** Incompetent lower esophageal sphincter

   Diminished strength of the lower esophageal sphincter makes it easier for food and fluid from the stomach to wash up into the lower esophagus. This can create problems with GERD. Decreased HCL production would actually alleviate some of the side effects of GERD.

79. **c.** Document them

   It is important that all information provided by a patient about their advance directives be documented, so there is a record of this information. While it is not necessary to check them with the family, it is important in most instances to have open communication with the family with the patient's consent.

80. **a.** Infection

   Decreases in immune function can heighten risk of infection in an older adult.

81. **d.** 85%

   Due to the high number of comorbid conditions, the incidence of pain in the nursing home is very high. More than half of older adults in nursing homes have osteoarthritis, in addition to other painful conditions.

82. **b.** Recognize excellence in practice

   Certification brings a recognition of excellence.

83. **b.** Delirium

   An acute change in cognition, particularly following surgery, is characteristic of delirium. There is no evidence in the stem of the question that the patient has been experiencing a gradual decline that would be characteristic of dementia.

84. **a.** Cherry angiomas, senile lentigines (liver spots), and skin tags

   While each of the other conditions can occur in older adults, these three conditions are characteristics of aging.

85. **a.** Written information describing the patient's desires for life-sustaining treatment

   The definition of a living will is written information about desires for life-sustaining treatment. Answer "b" is the definition of a durable power of attorney for health care.

86. **a.** Vaginal atrophy and dryness

   Vaginal atrophy and dryness are common changes of aging secondary to decreases in estrogen.

87. **d.** Smoking cessation

   Smoking cessation is an example of primary prevention because it is an intervention that can prevent the onset of illness.

88. **a.** Active lifestyle

   An active lifestyle can help prevent osteoporosis. The other answer choices can contribute to increased risk.

89. **c.** Renal dysfunction, neuropathy, and retinopathy

   Microvascular changes are often present in advance of other vascular problems. Organs that rely on the circulatory function of micro capillaries can be easily damaged.

90. **b.** Peripheral neuropathy

   Peripheral neuropathy is a common side effect of isoniazid. It can be managed through the use of B_6.

91. **b.** Developing cultural competence in the care of older adults

   Cultural competence is important to avoid the problems listed in the other answer responses.

92. **a.** Cerebrovascular disease

   Cerebrovascular disease is the most common cause of seizures in older adults. Although an electrolyte imbalance can also bring on a seizure it is not the most common cause.

93. **a.** MDS

    The MDS is the tool used for resident assessment in nursing homes. OASIS is used in home care.

94. **a.** Medication errors, falls, skin breakdown, and infection rates

    Medication errors, falls, skin breakdown, and infection rates are all areas sensitive to quality-improvement initiatives, and are important hallmarks of quality in long-term care.

95. **d.** Hyperresonance

    The increase in size will also increase resonance in this population.

96. **c.** Methotrexate, hydroxychloroquine (Plaquenil)

    These medications should be recognized as first-line disease-modifying drugs for RA. Tylenol, Percocet, and Aleve are analgesic medications. Phenobarbital is an antiseizure medication. Elavil and Prozac are antidepressant medications.

97. **c.** Glaucoma

    Glaucoma tends to have very few signs and symptoms, which is why ocular pressure should be checked regularly. One of the signs with may be present is the presence of colored rings around lights. As an aside, the presence of colored halos around objects is often considered a sign of digoxin toxicity.

98. **a.** Orthopnea

    The most common direct causes of increased pressure ulcer risk are moisture, shearing, and inactivity. Orthopnea might indirectly increase risk, but only if a person has one of these additional risk factors.

99. **d.** "Are you able to dress yourself?"

    A functional assessment includes an assessment of a patient's mobility and transfer skills, as well as their ability to perform activities of daily living such as bathing, dressing, and grooming.

100. **b.** Chronic lymphocytic leukemia

    Chronic lymphocytic leukemia is the most common leukemia in older adults, whereas acute lymphocytic leukemia is the most common leukemia in children.

101. **a.** Measure an attribute consistently

    A reliable tool is one that measures the same attribute consistently each and every time it is used.

102. **b.** Faces Pain Scale

The Faces Pain Scale is a valid and reliable tool to measure pain in older adults.

103. **d.** Constipation

The risk of constipation increases with age. Certain medications, such as opiates, tricyclic antidepressants, and anticholinergics, increase this risk further.

104. **c.** Decreased peripheral circulation

Decreases in peripheral circulation can prevent rewarming of the extremities. This can increase the risk of hypothermia. It is important to note that hypothermia may not only be a risk during cold temperatures, but also during prolonged surgical procedures.

105. **b.** Measuring the number of patients who had falls in their bedrooms

An outcomes audit looks at the impact of interventions. An example of one type of outcome that they might measure is the impact on patient falls.

106. **c.** 1960s

In the early 1960s, Laurie Gunther suggested that nurses required more science on which to base their practice.

107. **c.** 18.5 to 24.9

A normal BMI for an older adult is considered to be 18.5 to 24.9, which is the same as for younger people. Older adults with a BMI below 18.5 have a higher risk of mortality. Interestingly, there is some evidence to suggest that a slightly higher BMI will convey a mortality advantage in some older adults.

108. **a.** Fever and increased white blood cell count

Older adults tend to lack the characteristic symptoms of infection, including fever and increased white blood count. The other answer options are not signs or symptoms of infection in either older or younger patients.

109. **a.** Take extra time to adapt to the dim light before trying to find a seat

Older eyes take longer to adjust to changing light conditions. Moving from an area of light to dark can increase risk of falls. They should take time to adapt before finding a seat.

110. **b.** Assessment

Like all nursing diagnoses, those related to spirituality are no different. The beginning of the care plan begins with an assessment.

111. **a.** Medicare

    Medicare is the largest primary source of payment for the medical care of older adults.

112. **b.** Pneumonia and atelectasis

    The incidence of both pneumonia and atelectasis are increased in this population because of normal changes that take place in the respiratory system.

113. **b.** A decrease in bladder muscle tone, which results in a lessened ability to postpone voiding.

    Older adults tend to have decreased bladder capacity, increases in residual volume, and decreased perception of the need to void.

114. **b.** Perform orthostatic blood pressure and pulse assessment

    If the patient is reporting dizziness with standing, it is possible that they are experiencing orthostatic hypotension. An orthostatic assessment should be performed. A low-sodium diet could further exacerbate hypotension.

115. **c.** 75%

    The vast majority of hospice patients are older adults, but certainly not all patients. Other age groups are represented in smaller proportions.

116. **c.** Older American Resources and Services Assessment

    This tool allows service providers to determine the impact of a variety of care services on the functional status of older adults.

117. **d.** Erythema, edema, ulceration

    The redness, particularly nonblanchable redness, is the hallmark characteristic.

118. **c.** Rotator cuff tendonitis

    It could be reasoned that the inflammation from the tendonitis caused the impingement.

119. **c.** Beneficence

    Practitioners often struggle with the balance of beneficence (doing good) and nonmaleficence (doing no harm). Practitioners should first seek to do no harm.

120. **a.** Presbycusis

    Age-related hearing loss (presbycusis) is the cumulative effect of aging on hearing, and the most common cause of hearing loss in older adults.

121. **b.** Loss of sphincter control

Loss of sphincter control can lead to incontinence. Older adults tend to have decreased peristalsis.

122. **b.** To stabilize his vital signs and give fluid resuscitation

The first concern is to ensure patient safety. A patient with a social history that can cause significant liver damage is at substantial risk of severe bleeding. Stabilization of vital signs is the priority.

123. **b.** Nurses and health care professionals fail to detect problem alcohol use

Often an assessment of alcohol use is not performed. Standardized tools such as the CAGE can be used to help assess problematic use.

124. **a.** Cimetidine (Tagamet)

Cimetidine (Tagamet) is an example of an H_2 receptor blocker. Fexofenadine (Allegra), on the other hand, is an example of an H_1 receptor blocker.

125. **d.** It was the first federal health care legislation to be broadly supported by the American Medical Association

The American Medical Association voiced strong opposition to the enactment of Medicare legislation in the 1950s and 1960s.

126. **b.** Continue for some years to come

The growth in the numbers of older adults will continue as baby boomers hit their senior years.

127. **b.** Brain natriuretic peptide and complete chemistry profile

BNP levels can be used to rule out acute heart failure. Blood chemistry results will help uncover other causes of heart failure. CA-125 is a cancer marker. C-reactive protein is a marker for inflammation. ANA is a test for antinuclear antibodies, primarily used to detect autoimmune problems.

128. **b.** Once a day

Lantus is a long-acting insulin. It should be administered once daily.

129. **b.** Cardiovascular dysfunction

Cardiovascular dysfunction is one of the most common underlying causes of erectile dysfunction (ED). In addition, many medications used to treat hypertension also can cause ED.

130. **a.** Poor nutrition

Malnutrition is a common cause of folate deficiency anemia. Folate is found in the greatest quantities in enriched foods, such as breads and cereals.

131. **d.** Respite care

Respite care refers to a temporary placement, often in a nursing home, in order to give a caregiver a break from the strain of daily caregiving.

132. **c.** A number of chronic illnesses affect the sexual function of the elderly

Impotence is not considered to be a normal change of aging. Men older than 75, and in some instances men in their 90s, father children.

133. **b.** The patients can declare their desires regarding end-of-life care

Requiring patients to provide advance directives allows patients to state their desires about end of life care.

134. **c.** Acute exacerbations of their asthma

Respiratory viruses create additional concern for all patients with asthma, as they can cause acute exacerbations of asthma.

135. **c.** Hypothyroidism

Characteristic signs of hypothyroidism include weight gain, bradycardia, fatigue, and intolerance to cold.

136. **c.** She is Asian

Risk factors for osteoporosis include being female, postmenopausal, being of Caucasian or Asian descent, having small stature, lack of weight-bearing activity, previous fracture.

137. **c.** Blocks the action of angiotensin II

Medications to treat hypertension do not cure or prevent disease. The specific action of losartan (Cozaar) is to block the receptors for angiotensin II.

138. **b.** Depression, dementia, urinary function, and health literacy

Each of these issues might be covered in a nursing assessment.

139. **b.** Changes in senses of smell and taste

The only normal change of aging listed relates to smell and taste. The other changes listed should not be considered normal and should be followed up with additional evaluation.

140. **b.** Paranoia

Paranoia is an anxiety-laden thought process in which a patient may fear others are attempting to harm them.

141. **b.** Noncompliant

Nonadherence or noncompliance can be a problem for patients who are

142. **b.** An organized system of beliefs, practices, and rituals designed to foster closeness to a sacred reality

143. **c.** Have one nurse volunteer to develop and teach the wound care after learning it from a wound care consultant who is familiar with the procedure.

    Developing a mentorship model is an excellent approach. It is cost-effective and fosters collegiality.

144. **c.** Failure to thrive

    Failure to thrive is often the term given when a patient experiences frailty, malnutrition, and weight loss without a physiological explanation.

145. **a.** Aortic stenosis

    Aortic stenosis is the only murmur heard during the systolic phase. Aortic regurgitation and mitral stenosis are diastolic murmurs.

146. **b.** Seborrheic keratosis

    Seborrheic keratosis are large, brown lesions that have a "stuck-on" appearance.

147. **a.** Measure an attribute consistently

    A tool that is highly reliable and highly consistent. Note that this is different than being valid.

148. **a.** Increased levels of collagen

    As people age, increased levels of collagen can build up in endothelial walls. This collagen can trap glucose, further narrowing vessels.

149. **a.** Insulin will provide the quickest way to reach the optimum glycemic target for you.

    Oral medications are traditionally the first line of treatment for type 2 diabetes, except in the case of extreme high blood sugar. In this instance, insulin will help stabilize blood sugar levels more quickly than oral medications.

150. **d.** Onset of delirium

    The onset of delirium in a newly admitted hospital patient is an ominous sign. Hospitalized patients who develop delirium are more than twice as likely to die or require new nursing home placement than those who do not.

151. **c.** Pharmacodynamics

of drugs. Pharmacodynamics center on the movement of medications through the body and pharmacogenomics are focused on gene–medication interactions.

152. **b.** Detached retina

The signs indicating that this is a detached retina are that it only occurred acutely in one eye following a bumpy morning on the golf course.

153. **d.** All of the above

Palliative care is specialized medical care for people with serious illnesses. It focuses on providing patients with relief from both the physical and psychological symptoms and stress of a serious illness. Its goal is to provide quality of life for both the patient and the family.

154. **d.** *Klebsiella pneumoniae*

Klebsiella is most common in persons who are immunosuppressed.

155. **c.** Condoms may be used to protect older adults against STIs.

Condoms may be used to protect against sexually transmitted infections across the life span.

156. **b.** Blurred vision and difficulty reading

Macular degeneration often causes vision to become distorted in the center of the visual field, sometimes preserving vision in the periphery. The center-field distortions can make reading particularly difficult.

157. **c.** High blood cholesterol level

Cholesterol levels below 200 are desirable. Levels 200 to 239 are considered borderline. Levels of 240 or higher are considered high.

158. **c.** Inspection, palpation, percussion, and auscultation

A respiratory assessment of an older adult should include all facets of assessment, just as in a younger adult.

159. **c.** Shortness of breath, fatigue, or epigastric discomfort

Older adults often do not present with severe chest pain when having an infarction. Common signs include shortness of breath, fatigue, and/or epigastric discomfort.

160. **d.** Assess Mr. L's preferred method of communication

The nurse should simply assess the preferred method of communication. This may be different for each patient. This can also help open a discussion about the need for assistive devices, such as

161. **b.** Sociological

When thinking of disengagement theory, it is understood that this relates to the relationship of the older adult to society at large. Therefore, this is considered a sociological theory.

162. **d.** National Council of State Boards of Nursing

The Five Rights of Delegation were identified in *Delegation: Concepts and Decision-Making Process* and can be used as a mental checklist to assist nurses in multiple roles to clarify the critical elements of the decision-making process.

163. **c.** Both a and b

Older adults often have difficulty with both falling asleep and staying asleep.

164. **a.** Is reversible/medications

It is important that family members learn that delirium is both common and reversible in older adults. Unlike dementia, delirium will resolve, usually prior to discharge.

165. **d.** A low-level type of care in which the emphasis is on doing to the patient rather that working with the patient

Be sure to pay careful attention to words like *except* in the stem of the question.

166. **b.** Nuts, liver, and green leafy vegetables

In addition to foods that are fortified with folic acid, these foods are all naturally high in folic acid.

167. **b.** Quality improvement

Quality-assessment committees often direct and oversee initiatives to improve quality-of-care indicators within institutions.

168. **c.** "You have excess uric acid, which creates deposits of urate crystals in the soft tissue surrounding your peripheral joints."

Gout is an inborn error of purine metabolism. As GFR decreases with age, older adults are less able to excrete uric acid from their bodies leading to an excessive amount of uric acid. This acid can form crystals that cause painful attacks.

169. **c.** Delirium

A temporary change in cognitive status is delirium. Dementia has a slow, progressive onset. Confusion is a nonspecific term that can be applied to patients with either delirium or dementia.

170. **c.** Document why restraints are ordered, how they will be evaluated, and when they should be discontinued.

Orders for restraint use must be reviewed every 4 hours. Restraints must be released every 2 hours, and range-of-motion exercises should be performed on the restrained limb.

171. **c.** Anaphylaxis

These symptoms all indicate anaphylaxis. This should be considered a medical emergency.

172. **d.** Turn and reposition the patient every 1 to 2 hours.

Turning and repositioning every 2 hours is one of the most common and most effective ways to prevent pressure ulcers.

173. **b.** The tool measures what it is intended to measure

A valid measure is one that measures what it is intended to measure. An example might be a glucometer to measure glucose levels.

174. **a.** Can be caused by bladder muscle weakness

Incontinence can be caused by bladder muscle or pelvic floor weakness.

175. **a.** Rigidity, bradykinesia, and tremors

Rigidity, bradykinesia, and tremors are common signs of Parkinson's disease.

176. **b.** Omnibus Budget Reconciliation Act

OBRA 87 is largely responsible for the quality environment in which nursing homes operate today, including a more stringent survey process; revised care standards, sanctions, and remedies; training of nurse aides; and use of the Resident Assessment Instrument.

177. **c.** Increase

When there are low levels of protein in the blood, drugs do not have enough protein to bind to. Without these needed binding sites, the amount of free drug can rise. The problem is exacerbated with medications that are highly protein bound. In these cases, low albumin levels can cause drug toxicity.

178. **c.** Decrease in the production of estrogen

During menopause, estrogen levels decline. This is the cause of several changes that can occur with age, including decrease in breast size and decreased vaginal lubrication.

179. **a.** Arrange an appointment for him to see the physician.

   A mole that increases in size or has an irregular border or color should be evaluated by a physician.

180. **c.** 21%

   According to the U.S. Census Bureau, the population is expected to become much older, with nearly one in five U.S. residents age 65 and older in 2030, or approximately 21% of the total population.

181. **c.** Confusion

   Dysuria (a) and flank pain (d) are typical signs of a UTI. An atypical sign sometimes manifested by some older adults is confusion.

182. **b.** Herpes zoster

   The clue in the stem is that the rash is in a line, on only one side of the body. This is characteristic of herpes zoster, also known as shingles.

183. **a.** Dizziness

   Because timolol and metoprolol are both beta blockers, there may be an increased risk of blood pressure or heart rate problems. Any problems with dizziness should be reported.

184. **a.** Cost–benefit analysis

   A cost–benefit analysis is a framework used to assess whether a particular health care intervention is worthwhile; or how the cost of the intervention compares to the benefits of patient health and well-being.

185. **d.** Restorative

   A restraint cannot restore health or function. There is no such thing as a "restorative" restraint.

186. **b.** Altered cognitive status

   Lack of privacy, decreased bulk in diet (including decreased availability of fresh fruits and vegetables), and decreased bowel peristalsis can all contribute to constipation.

187. **c.** Pain and discomfort when urinating

   Classic signs of a UTI include pain and discomfort while urinating.

188. **b.** Drug allergies

   The presence of drug allergies is important to address in each patient.

189. **a.** History of seizures

     Patients with a history of seizures should avoid this medication since it may increase the risk of seizures.

190. **b.** Disorder of the substantia nigra that decreases ability to initiate movement

     Part of the Parkinson's disease process develops as cells are destroyed in certain parts of the brainstem, particularly the crescent-shaped cell mass known as the substantia nigra.

191. **a.** Anticonvulsants

     Traditional analgesics do little to ease the pain of postherpic neuralgia. Anticonvulsants work to quiet the neurological signaling at the root of the problem.

192. **c.** Decreased passage of oxygen from the alveoli to the blood

     Thickening of the pulmonary tissue, which occurs with age, decreases the ability of oxygen to pass through the lung tissue and into the blood.

193. **a.** Assist with career goal accomplishment

     Mentoring is one of the most effective ways to guide the new nurse through the process of developing and accomplishing long- and short-term career goals.

194. **a.** State's Nurse Practice Act

     All states and territories have enacted a Nurse Practice Act (NPA) by the state's legislature. Each NPA establishes a board of nursing (BON) that has the authority to develop administrative rules or regulations to clarify nurses' scope of practice.

195. **a.** Use less soap because it is drying, keep well hydrated, apply emollient cream

     Overuse of soap is particularly drying to older skin. The most common treatment for dry skin is the use of moisturizers to reduce water loss and soothe the skin. Hydration and the use of humidifiers is also helpful.

196. **b.** 50%

     Studies have shown that, on average, around 50% of older adults are noncompliant with medical treatment plans due to multiple factors (e.g., overall complexity of treatment plan; multiple medications)

197. **b.** Heart failure

     The presence of pedal edema, rales, shortness of breath, confusion, and recent history of weight gain are all characteristic of heart failure.

198. **a.** Increased income

Typically, older adults choose to move from one environment to another for several different health, financial, and social reasons.

199. **d.** Psychosocial

Gerotranscendence characterizes transitions into older adulthood as a normal part of human development, viewing older adulthood as a developmental stage.

200. **a.** UTI

A new onset of cognitive change is a common sign of UTI in older adults.

201. **c.** Bony prominences

Bony prominences are considered particularly at risk for the development of pressure ulcers. The sacrum, coccyx, and heels are among the more common areas affected.

202. **c.** Focused history and physical exam as well as a review of functional ability and medications

203. **b.** Diminished T cell responsiveness

With aging, changes in helper T cells' ability to function cause a decreased cellular immune response in older adults, which makes them more susceptible to infections.

204. **c.** Onychomycosis

Onychomycosis is a fungal infection of the nail bed. Tinea pedis is commonly known as "athletes foot." Tinea versicolor is a yeast infection of the skin. Balanitis is an inflammation of the head of the penis.

205. **b.** Daytime napping of many older adults seems to compensate for night time sleep disturbances

Difficulty with sleep quality is common as people age. Short daytime napping can sometimes ameliorate fatigue caused by disturbed sleep patterns.

206. **b.** Control group

The experimental group is typically the group that receives an intervention. The control group typically does not.

207. **b.** A grayish arc surrounding the cornea

These lipid deposits are often called the "arcus senilis." They have no effect on vision and are considered harmless.

208. **a.** Medicare

   In the United States, Medicare is a national social insurance program, administered by the U.S. federal government since 1966. Medicare provides health insurance for Americans age 65 and older who have worked and paid into the system.

209. **b.** Some medications

   The categories that can affect GFR are substantial. In addition to NSAIDs, any medication that decreases blood pressure, or heart rate (beta blockers), affects the functioning of the kidney.

210. **c.** Infections, smoking, medications

   Infections, particularly those that affect smell (congestion) can also affect taste. Smoking and medications (such as chemotherapeutic agents) also change taste sensations.

211. **d.** Previous history of a fall

   The greatest risk factor for a fall is a history of a fall.

212. **d.** Exercise the involved joints regularly

   Although the tendency might be to want to rest these joints, just the opposite should occur. Patients with osteoarthritis should continue to move their joints regularly.

213. **a.** Information disclosure, access to emergency services, and participation in treatment decisions

   The Consumer Bill of Rights and Responsibilities that was adopted by the U.S. Advisory Commission on Consumer Protection and Quality in the Health Care Industry in 1998 mandates, among other rights, information disclosure, access to emergency services, and taking part in treatment decisions.

214. **c.** *Helicobacter pylori*

   GERD may be related to the presence of the bacteria *Helicobacter pylori*.

215. **a.** Exercising regularly every day, losing weight, stopping smoking

   Because this is a prediabetic patient, insulin and palliative care would not be indicated. Prediabetic patients should be on a low-fat diet. Most important, regular exercise, losing weight, and stopping smoking are going to be critical to prevent progression of the disease.

216. **d.** 10 seconds

   The timed Up-and-Go test examines the ability of a person to rise from a chair. For older adults, scores of 30 seconds or more indicate increased

217. **b.** Oxybutynin (Ditropan)

Oxybutynin (Ditropan) is an anticholinergic medication. Common side effects of anticholinergic medications are dry mouth and constipation.

218. **d.** "There are medications that would dilate the small vessels in your hands and fingers, but these drugs would dilate other vessels, too, which could cause harm."

The overall health and well-being of the patient needs to be considered in any potential treatment decision.

219. **b.** The safety culture of the institution

The IOM reports on the quality and safety of hospitals. Following IOM guidelines will aid improving the safety culture of the institution.

220. **a.** Cognitive status

Because the chief complaint is memory loss, an evaluation of cognitive status is in order. This would be followed by an attempt to rule out other problems that could be the cause of acute memory problems, such as infection. It should be noted again, that older adults often do not manifest a fever as a response to an infection.

221. **a.** Weakened vertebrae cause disk compression

As people age there can be an imbalance in the activity of osteoclasts and osteoblasts. The osteoblasts build bone, and this activity may diminish. The osteoclasts break down bone and this activity may increase in relationship to the osteoblasts. This imbalance, in conjunction with decreased estrogen levels, can lead to osteoporosis. The weakened vertebrae can become compressed leading to diminished stature.

222. **c.** Palliative

The main goal of palliative care is to provide symptom palliation. There is no goal to restore, rehabilitate, or cure.

223. **d.** Provide information on patient's wishes at the end of life

An advance directive provides information about a patient's wishes at the end of life.

224. **c.** The Joint Commission

The Joint Commission was previously known as the Joint Commission on Accreditation of Healthcare Organizations (JCAHO) and prior to that, as the Joint Commission on Accreditation of Hospitals (JCAH). This organization is responsible for the accreditation of both hospitals and nursing homes.

225. a. The patient develops confusion or exhibits a change in mental status

A change in mental status may indicate poor perfusion of oxygen to the brain. Further assessment should be performed.

226. a. Primary

Good nutrition is typically thought of as primary prevention. Once a disease develops, additional nutritional interventions may be needed to help prevent disease progression.

227. a. Biological

The Hayflick theory is a theory of aging that suggests that cells will continue to divide until they stop. With each cellular division the telomeres at the end of the cell shorten, indicating aging cells.

228. a. Renal dialysis every other day

Increased serum iron ferritin in the context of decreased iron and decreased total iron binding capacity are very common for patients undergoing renal dialysis.

229. c. Beta blockers

Beta blockers can decrease heart rate and diminish cardiac output.

230. c. Katz Index

The Katz Index is a measure of functional status. The Beers criteria are a set of guidelines for appropriate prescribing of medications. The Mini-Mental State Exam addresses cognitive function.

231. c. Dizziness and lightheadedness

The presence of dizziness and lightheadedness can predispose an older adult to a fall. These symptoms should be assessed following a change in position.

232. b. Medicaid

Medicare is funded by the federal government. Medicaid is funded by the states.

233. d. Cerumen impaction

Cerumen (earwax) impaction is a common cause of reduced hearing in older adults. As people age the earwax can become harder and more difficult to remove.

234. d. Hips and knees

Osteoarthritis commonly causes problems in the hips and knees.

235. **b.** Corn

   Corns are areas of thickened skin that develop on the top part of the foot to protect that area from irritation. They occur when something rubs against the foot repeatedly or causes excess pressure against part of the foot.

236. **c.** Quantitative research

   Because the researcher is looking at variables that can be quantified (pain level and number of pain medications given), this is quantitative research.

237. **a.** Fine-needle biopsy

   The first step of the assessment is to gather more information about the lump through a fine-needle biopsy.

238. **c.** Provide patients the opportunity to develop advance directives

   The requirement is simply that hospitals provide this opportunity to all patients. As a result, patients may or may not have advance directives.

239. **c.** Medications

   Medications are a common cause of delirium. After surgery, anesthetics, analgesics, and anticholinergic medications commonly cause delirium.

240. **b.** Discomfort, hurting, aching

   If an older adult is reluctant to report "pain" it may be helpful to ask if there is any discomfort, hurting, or aching.

241. **a.** Primary

   Immunizations are considered primary prevention as they are intended to prevent the onset of illness.

242. **a.** Intake and output, mucous membrane moisture, and urine specific gravity

   Intake and output, mucous membrane moisture, and urine specific gravity are all good indicators of hydration status in older adults. Although thirst is used in younger adults, it is not a reliable indicator in older adults due to changes in the thirst sensation.

243. **b.** Names a person for making health care decisions

   A durable power of attorney names a person who can make decisions for you if you are to become incapacitated. There may be separate powers of attorney for health care as well as for finances.

244. **c.** An aged person has a longer story to tell

Older adults have longer health histories than younger people because, quite simply, there is more history to review.

245. **c.** Psychological

The idea of self-actualization comes from Maslow's hierarchy of needs in which self-actualization is the final stage.

246. **b.** Decreasing osteoblast function

Changes in estrogen levels affect the balance of osteoclasts to osteoblasts. Remember that osteoclasts tear down bone, whereas osteoblasts build bone.

247. **c.** T cells

Older adults experience an overall decline in immunological capabilities. T cells are particularly affected by this change.

248. **c.** Polypharmacy

Polypharmacy is the use of multiple medications in older adults. Many sources define polypharmacy as the concurrent use of more than four medications.

249. **c.** Pneumonia

Normal changes of aging make an older adult more susceptible to pneumonia.

250. **b.** A duodenal ulcer

One of the key differences between a peptic ulcer and a duodenal ulcer is that a duodenal ulcer is relieved by eating food.

251. **b.** Qualitative research

Qualitative research generally involves the collection of text, narratives, and field notes as data. Using a focus group is a type of qualitative research.

252. **d.** Rising Medicare costs

Diagnostic related groups were an attempt to control costs.

253. **b.** Acetaminophen (Tylenol)

Tylenol is often used in older adults because it tends to have few drug interactions.

254. **b.** Zoloft

Zoloft is the only medication that blocks the reabsorption of serotonin. Elavil is a tricyclic antidepressant. Haldol is an antipsychotic. Restoril is a benzodiazepine.

255. **c.** Fewer alveoli

The number of alveoli remain constant, but with age the thoracic cage stiffens, there are fewer cilia, and a decreased cough reflex is seen.

256. **b.** Secondary

PSA screening is an example of secondary prevention because the goal is to diagnose and treat a disease (prostate cancer) earlier.

257. **a.** UTI

Confusion is a common manifestation of infection in older adults.

258. **b.** Sociological

The activity theory states that successful aging is partly defined by staying active and maintaining social connections.

259. **b.** Gait disturbance, dizziness, impaired concentration

Opioids can have several side effects that are more pronounced in older adults. These are gait disturbance, dizziness, and impaired concentration.

260. **a.** Live and die with dignity

Hospice allows people to live and die with dignity. Pain and other symptom management are critical; however, mental alertness is typically impaired at the end of life.

261. **b.** Polyuria, urinary urgency, increased frequency

BPH can prevent the bladder from emptying fully when voiding. Patients experience polyuria, urgency, and increased frequency. Dysuria, or painful urination, is not typical of BPH, but can instead signal a UTI.

262. **b.** Lack of standards

Standardized assessments should be used for older adults. Hopefully, you have learned the names of several standardized assessments for older adults.

263. **a.** The entire staff is involved in any decision making regarding the change

Change theory indicates that it is the staff who are critical in participating fully in any changes that need to be made.

264. **d.** Depression, anxiety, sleep disturbance

Untreated pain in older adults has several important consequences including depression, anxiety, and sleep disturbance.

265. **a.** Pregnant women, infants, people who are immunocompromised

Shingles can be contagious. It is important that women who are pregnant, people who have not had chicken pox, and people who are immunocompromised avoid contact with a person with shingles.

266. **a.** Headache, seizures, vomiting

Headache, seizures, and vomiting are all signs of the increased intracranial pressure, which would occur as a result of the subarachnoid hemorrhage.

267. **b.** Benadryl

Benadryl has strong anticholinergic side effects and a long half-life. It is a Beers Criteria medication that should generally be avoided in older adults.

268. **d.** Arrange a psychiatric consult for evaluation of her depression and treatment

A patient who screens positive on the GDS should be referred for follow-up for further evaluation and treatment.

269. **b.** A natural part of life

Hospice philosophy includes the idea that death is a natural part of life.

270. **a.** Sister Callista Roy

Roy is credited with the adaptation theory, which includes the idea that each individual is an interrelated set of biological, psychological, and social functions.

271. **b.** Secondary

Diagnostic tests generally fall under the category of secondary prevention.

272. **c.** 80%

Medicare typically covers 80% of reasonable and customary charges.

273. **d.** Passive neglect

Although active neglect refers to the active and intentional withholding of care from an older adult, passive neglect refers to the inability to provide basic care.

274. **a.** Salt and sugar

It is important to know that the taste for salt and sugar diminishes with age, leading older adults to overuse these ingredients. This is a particular problem for older adults with diabetes and hypertension.

275. **a.** Blood pressure and pulse while lying, sitting, and standing

Testing for orthostatic hypotension involves testing a person's blood pressure while he or she is lying, sitting, and standing. Assessment of pulse will determine if there is a rise in pulse rate to compensate for the reduction in blood pressure.

276. **a.** Dislocation of the prosthesis

Following hip replacement surgery there is a concern about dislocation of the prosthesis. For this reason patients are advised to avoid crossing their legs and avoid bending down (hip flexion). When sitting, the knees should be kept lower than the hips.

277. **a.** Integumentary system changes

These are all common changes in the integumentary system. There are decreases in elastin and subcutaneous fat, decreases in the number of sweat and sebaceous glands, and decreased vascular flow to the skin.

278. **d.** The family's grieving process is complete

The care of the terminally ill patient should also encompass the care of the family.

279. **b.** Delirium

Delirium is a common complication following surgery in older adults. It is characterized by having an acute onset and a limited duration.

280. **b.** Risedronate (Actonel)

Risedronate (Actonel) is an osteoclast inhibitor. By inhibiting osteoclast activity, bone mass can be restored.

281. **b.** Mental status for confusion or disorientation

When leaving medications at the bedside for self-administration (with the requisite facility permissions), a nurse should always confirm that a patient is cognitively intact and capable of self-administration.

282. **b.** Systolic blood pressure decrease of 20 mmHg and a diastolic blood pressure decrease of 10 mmHg after a position change

Orthostatic hypotension involves a drop of 20 mmHg, or a decrease of 10 mmHg when changing position. In older adults, the cause is often either hypovolemia or medication.

283. **c.** American Nurses Association

The *Code of Ethics for Nurses* was developed by the American Nurses Association as a guide for carrying out nursing responsibilities in a manner consistent with quality in nursing care and the ethical obligations of the profession.

284. **c.** A decline

Although a decline in erectile function is considered a normal change of aging, a loss of erectile function is a medical problem that can be treated.

285. **d.** Balding in patches

Although men may experience an overall decline in the amount of hair on their heads, the presence of bald patches is not considered normal.

286. **b.** Is a progressive conductive hearing loss that commonly occurs with age

Presbycusis is a form of hearing loss that occurs with age. It typically affects the ability of a person to hear high-frequency sounds.

287. **a.** Heartburn after a big meal or when lying supine

While people with hiatal hernia are often asymptomatic, when symptoms are present they can often mimic those of GERD.

288. **c.** Explain to Mr. Carter that this is a normal age-related change that occurs in the eye

The question describes an arcus senilis, a normal change of aging that requires no intervention.

289. **b.** Stress/Kegel exercises

Stress incontinence is caused by the bladder leaking urine during physical activity or exertion. Kegel exercises can keep the muscles around the urethra strong and working well. Urinary incontinence is much more common in older adults.

290. **a.** Using an active listening approach to communication

Good communication strategies around the death of a patient are those that can encourage family members to share and process their feelings. Stating that the patient died a "good death" can shut down communication.

291. **c.** Open questioning, acknowledging, and summarizing

Open questioning, acknowledging, and summarizing allow the listener to know that you have heard what they are saying.

292. d. Dame Cicely Saunders

Dame Cicely Saunders is often credited with being the founder of modern hospice.

293. d. Dorothea Orem

Dorothea Orem is credited with the theory of self-care. Through the lens of this theory the nurse is thought to be a person who helps patients care for themselves.

294. c. Decreased respiratory muscle strength, decreased airway and lung compliance

Decreased respiratory muscle strength, decreased airway and lung compliance can all make artificial ventilation more difficult. Older adults have decreased vital capacity.

295. c. Dementia

Lewy body dementia is a form of cognitive impairment characterized by gradual cognitive decline. It is sometimes associated with Parkinson's disease.

296. c. Tertiary

A speech–language pathologist can help minimize speech and language problems, often following a stroke. This would therefore be a form of tertiary prevention.

297. a. Medicare Part A

Hospital care is funded under Part A, outpatient services are covered under Part B, prescription medications are covered under Part D.

298. d. Bone reabsorption causes the bone to lose calcium and decreases the ability to produce material for the bone matrix

Height will decrease, often as a result of a shortening of the spinal column. Muscle mass and strength decrease.

299. a. Posttraumatic stress disorder

Older adults experiencing abuse are at risk of posttraumatic stress disorder in the same way that younger abuse victims are.

300. a. Muscular pain from overuse

The lack of cardiac symptoms combined with the patient history of overuse, indicate that the pain is muscular in origin. While a shoulder can be dislocated, a rotator cuff cannot.

301. a. Polypharmacy

Polypharmacy generally refers to taking four or more medications simultaneously.

302. d. Transactional leadership

The focus on the unit is centered on completing tasks that a manager has put in place. The manager will measure performance based on the completion of these tasks, therefore the nurses will make them a priority. This is an example of transactional leadership.

303. b. When the kidneys are not functioning properly, drugs tend to remain in the bloodstream longer, increasing the risk of drug toxicity

304. b. Optimal patient outcomes, access to services, and cost-effectiveness

An organization that implements a QI program experiences benefits such as improved patient health, increased access to services, and avoidance of costs associated with process failures, errors, or poor outcomes.

305. d. All of the above

Hospice care can take place in various settings, including the home, hospital, and long-term care facility.

306. d. The secretions of the salivary glands diminish

Losing teeth is not a normal change of aging. Incidence of hiatal hernia will increase with age. This is also not a normal change of aging. Pertussis is also known as whooping cough, a respiratory condition.

307. a. Absorption

The way drugs move into the body is called absorption. The movement through the tissues is distribution. Metabolism is the breakdown of drugs. Excretion is the movement of drugs out of the body.

308. c. Central vision loss

Macular degeneration can result in central vision loss.

309. c. Neutropenia, anemia, and thrombocytopenia

The term *pancytopenia* means that all blood cell lines are affected, including the white blood cells (neutropenia), the red blood cells (anemia), and the platelets (thrombocytopenia).

310. b. The movement of drugs within the body

Pharmacokinetics refers to the movement of drugs within the body.

311. **c.** Erythropoietin (Epogen)

Patients with chronic renal disease are unable to produce their own erythropoietin to stimulate red blood cell formation. Therefore, synthetic erythropoietin (Epogen) is used to stimulate the production of red blood cells and prevent anemia.

312. **a.** Smoking since the age of 18

Smoking is the number one cause of COPD. Other causes can include air pollution and genetic disorders.

313. **b.** Hildegard Peplau

Peplau is known for the middle range theory of interpersonal relations.

314. **c.** A "good death"

The goal of palliative care is to provide symptom palliation and ultimately, a "good death."

315. **b.** Essential tremor

An essential tremor is one that is exacerbated with movement.

316. **c.** Hypermagnesemia

Frequent ingestion of magnesium-containing antacids can result in hypermagnesemia (high levels of magnesium).

317. **b.** Hypothyroidism

The incidence of hypothyroidism increases with age.

318. **a.** The GDS

The GDS is a common tool for assessing depression in older adults. The Beck Depression Inventory is another commonly used tool.

319. **d.** The patient becomes short of breath when ambulating to the bathroom

Dyspnea upon exertion is a common manifestation of COPD. For this reason many patients with COPD require supplemental oxygen as the disease progresses.

320. **b.** Decreased sensitivity to insulin

Older adults may have decreases in their sensitivity to insulin, particularly in the context of having increases in body mass index (BMI).

321. **b.** Alcohol use

The CAGE screening tool asks about at-risk drinking behaviors.

322. **b.** Evidence-based practice

The goal of evidence-based practice is the integration of clinical expertise/expert opinion, external scientific evidence from the literature, and client/patient/caregiver perspectives to provide high-quality patient care.

323. **b.** Electrolyte imbalance

Patients with end stage renal disease are at high risk of electrolyte imbalances as well as fluid retention.

324. **a.** Stop eating grapefruit and drinking grapefruit juice

Grapefruit and grapefruit juice can affect the metabolism of many medications, including statins and cardiac medications.

325. **b.** Drug sensitivity

Older adults are much more sensitive to medications than younger adults. For this reason, gerontologists use the maxim, "start low and go slow" when referring to the method of determining appropriate dosing for older adults.

326. **d.** None of the above

Older adults typically will have their hospital stays covered by Medicare. The length of stay is expected to be, on average, longer than a younger adult.

327. **b.** Someone living past 110

A supercentenarian is someone who has lived to or passed his or her 110th birthday. This age is achieved by about 1 in 1,000 persons.

328. **a.** Faith practices tend to remain relatively stable over time

It is a common myth that older adults become more religious as they age. Typically faith practices are relatively stable over time.

329. **a.** Stochastic

Stochastic theories are a form of biological theory, which points to the way genetic damage accumulates in DNA over time.

330. **c.** Call 911

You should recognize this as a sign of a stroke and call 911.

331. **b.** He will likely need to go to a nursing home for rehabilitation

Stroke recovery can be lengthy, peak recovery may take 3 to 6 months following a stroke. During this time intensive nursing care and physical therapy are needed. Therefore, this recovery often takes place in a

332. **b.** The older adults ranging in age from 65 to 100+ were too diverse to be grouped into one category

It is important to recognize the tremendous diversity in the age range of people who are typically included in the group "older adults." There is as much of a difference between a 30-year-old and a 60-year-old as there is between a 60-year-old and a 90-year-old.

333. **d.** Address the older adult by his or her last name until instructed to do otherwise

Avoid using terms like honey and sweetie. These terms are disrespectful. Older adults should always be addressed by their last names, unless they suggest otherwise. Speaking slightly louder and with a slightly lower tone of voice can be helpful.

334. **d.** Constipation can contribute to incontinence

Older adults experiencing incontinence should not limit their fluid intake, as this can lead to dehydration. Urinary incontinence should not be considered a normal change of aging. Efforts should be made to address underlying causes, such as pelvic floor weakness. Constipation can contribute to incontinence.

335. **a.** Do an oral health assessment to determine whether oral health problems are contributing to her weight loss

Other interventions, such as ordering larger portion sizes, will not be effective if there are physical problems affecting her ability to eat. When at all possible, real food should be used to help stave off weight loss, instead of supplements.

336. **a.** Nutrition

Nutrition is important for proper healing. Patients should ensure they are consuming a sufficient number of calories and taking in enough fluids to ensure adequate healing. For patients without underlying renal concerns, consuming adequate amounts of protein can aid healing.

337. **d.** There can be enormous diversity in every person at every age in every part of the body

It is important to recognize the diversity that occurs both naturally and through lifestyle choices, which can have an impact on all body systems.

338. **a.** Turn and reposition the patient every 2 hours

This classic intervention is perhaps the best way to prevent pressure ulcers in bedridden older adults with limited mobility.

339. **c.** Lack of fever does not mean lack of infection in older adults

Although the validity of oral temperatures can vary depending on the

older adult with a serious infection without a fever. While a temperature of 97 degree F is considered low, it is not unusual.

340. **c.** Loss of the ability to hear high-pitched frequencies

Thick, dry cerumen can be another reason for hearing difficulties in older adults. High-pitched ringing in the ears is called tinnitus. The inability to read small print is called presbyopia.

341. **a.** A breakdown in the absorption of intraocular fluid leading to an increase in intraocular pressure

Glaucoma is an eye disorder in which intraocular fluid builds up in the eye. This increased fluid creates increased pressure that can lead to loss of vision.

342. **d.** None of the above

Physical activity should be encouraged in older adults. Weight bearing exercise will help prevent osteoporosis. People with arthritis should be encouraged to continue to move their joints.

343. **d.** All of the above

There are many things that can affect the quality of sleep in older adults. These include dementia, depression, stress and anxiety, pain, medications, urinary incontinence, and chronic illness.

344. **d.** Social support

The SPICES assessment examines: sleep, problems with eating and feeding, incontinence, confusion, evidence of falls, and skin breakdown.

345. **c.** Unilateral weakness

Signs of a stroke include the FAST criteria:

Facial drooping: A section of the face, usually only on one side, that is drooping and hard to move

Arm weakness: The inability to raise one's arm fully

Speech difficulties: An inability or difficulty to understand or produce speech

Time: Time is of the essence when having a stroke, and an immediate call to emergency services or trip to the hospital is recommended

346. **d.** None of the above

Patients with GERD should eat smaller meals and avoid lying down following meals.

347. **a.** COPD

Although shortness of breath is a common symptom for all of these

348. **b.** "You should not stop taking them because you can lose your vision."

Patients with glaucoma often do not have any signs or symptoms. It is important for patients to know that even if they do not experience eye pain, they need to take their eye medications as prescribed in order to keep the intraocular pressure under control.

349. **a.** Dietary changes and weight-bearing exercise

Hormone replacement therapy should be avoided because it may increase the risk of certain cancers. Osteoclast inhibitors may be tried after diet and lifestyle changes have already been implemented.

350. **d.** Medicare D

The Part D benefit relates to prescription coverage. Part A is hospital insurance, Part B is medical insurance.

351. **a.** Use a validated tool such as the PAINAD

It is important to realize that standardized tools to measure pain in cognitively impaired older adults exists. These patients are particularly at risk of having untreated pain, because they are often unable to ask for pain medication.

352. **a.** A randomized controlled trial

A randomized controlled trial requires both random selection and random assignment to a group.

353. **b.** Deep vein thrombosis

We know it is not congestive heart failure, because the swelling would likely manifest in both legs for a patient with CHF. The location (the calf) rules out gout. The use of heparin rules out a fracture.

354. **d.** All of the above

Mrs. Johnson has numerous risk factors for acute-care constipation, including decreased movement, use of narcotic medications, and decreased intake of high-fiber foods.

355. **b.** They comprise the majority of patients on acute-care medical–surgical units.

Only about 29% of older adults live alone, and less than 5% live in nursing homes. They do, however, comprise the majority of hospitalized medical–surgical patients.

356. **b.** 1 in 5

By the year 2030, approximately 20% of the population, or one in five adults, will be older than age 65.

357. d. Women are more likely to live alone

In part because women outlive men, women are more likely to live alone.

358. b. Cultural diversity will increase over the next decade

As with the entire U.S. population, the diversity of older adults is increasing. We will expect to see increases in racial and ethnic diversity among older adults over the next decade and beyond.

359. b. Florida, Maine, West Virginia

Persons 65+ constituted approximately 15% or more of the total population in 11 states in 2011 with Florida, Maine, and West Virginia being the highest.

360. b. It increased the number of men receiving a college education

The GI bill provided financial incentives for veterans to return to college. This bill substantially increased the number of men with college educations in the current cohort of older adults.

361. c. She will be at an increased risk of falls when moving from bright light into darkness

Older adults have decreased visual accommodation. Because of this, they can be at increased risk of falls with rapid shifts in lighting.

362. c. As people age they can have decreased perception of salt

Generally speaking, older adults should avoid excessive sodium intake. However, at the same time they may seek to increase their intake of sodium due to decreased salt perception.

363. b. Coronary artery disease

Coronary artery disease is the number one cause of death among U.S. women.

364. d. All of the above

Arteriosclerosis causes narrowing of the arteries. This increases blood pressure and raises stroke risk.

365. b. Encourage the patient to exercise to the best of his or her ability

Patients with heart failure can still strengthen heart muscle and increase cardiac output through reasonable exercise regimens. They should limit sodium intake as this can put additional strain on the heart. Patients with heart failure should monitor their weight daily so that they can ensure they are not retaining too much fluid.

366. **b.** Programmed aging

Programmed aging is a theory of aging that states that life expectancy is predetermined and timed for individual species, with cells programmed to divide a certain number of times. Functional changes in the cells cause aging of the cells and thus the organism.

367. **a.** Wear and tear

The wear and tear theory of aging suggests that the effects of aging are caused by damage done to cells and body systems over time, essentially "wearing out" these cells and systems due to use. Once these cells "wear out" they can no longer function correctly.

368. **c.** Immunity theory

The immunity theory of aging professes that the rate of aging is largely controlled by the immune system. As the body ages, the number of critical cells in the immune system decreases and become less functional.

369. **a.** Free radical theory

The free radical theory of aging (FRTA) states that organisms age because cells accumulate free radical damage over time. For most biological structures, free radical damage is closely associated with oxidative stress damage to an organism.

370. **c.** Immunity theory

As people age, they undergo immunosenescence. The thymus, which produces T cells against new invaders, atrophies markedly after adolescence, and this decline results in a less robust immune response to bacteria, viruses, and presumably allergens.

371. **b.** Rheumatoid arthritis

Rheumatoid arthritis is a type of arthritis, more prevalent in women, which is characterized by exacerbations and remissions as well as severe joint deformities.

372. **d.** A low-fat, no-added-sugar, no-added-salt diet

Looking at the list of medications, it is clear that the patient has diabetes, hypertension, and hyperlipidemia. The presence of these conditions warrants a low-fat, no added sugar, no added salt diet.

373. **b.** They carry a higher risk of side effects in older adults.

374. **b.** Try increasing daytime activity by taking frequent walks

Increasing daytime activity can help expend energy. Sedatives should be avoided because they can increase confusion. Restraints should not be used for this purpose.

375. **a.** The Braden Scale

The Braden Scale is used to measure the risk of developing a pressure ulcer. The Tinetti Scale is used to assess fall risk. There is no such thing as the PURS.

376. **c.** Performance and continued improvement in care

The Joint Commission is responsible for accrediting both hospitals and long-term care institutions. An important standard is the continuous process of improving care.

377. **a.** Presbycusis

Presbycusis refers to the progressive loss of ability to hear high-pitched sounds. This hearing loss actually begins as early as the 20s and gradually progresses over time.

378. **c.** S_4

While the presence of S_4 is considered pathological in younger adults, it may be a normal finding in older adults. It results from the sound of blood moving into a slightly hypertrophic ventricle.

379. **c.** Changes in behavior, fatigue, and loss of appetite

Older adults are less likely to see large shifts in white blood cell counts and temperature. Instead, an older adult may experience fatigue, changes in behavior, and loss of appetite.

380. **a.** Tremor, palpitations, and proximal weakness

Signs of hyperthyroidism include tremor, palpitations, and weakness. Signs of hypothyroidism include fatigue, weight gain, and depression.

381. **c.** The heart valves stiffen and become thicker

An anticipated change of aging is that the heart valves will stiffen and become thicker.

382. **a.** Keep the wound clean and covered with a wet to moist dressing, begin a toileting program, and prevent the patient from putting pressure on the wound

Wet to dry dressings and peroxide should be avoided in healthy healing pressure ulcers. Establishing a toileting program will help prevent moisture from penetrating the wound and will help keep it clean. Measures must be taken to ensure that the patient does not put pressure on the wound.

383. **a.** Nursing grand theory

A nursing "grand theory" is a theory of nursing that attempts to define

384. **d.** All of the above

   Hospice care is centered on caring for the whole person, including the physical, psychological, and spiritual domains.

385. **c.** "Yes, there is a relationship between family history and dementia."

   There are specific genes that have been specifically linked to certain forms of dementia, including the APOE genotype linked to Alzheimer's disease.

386. **d.** Medigap

   Medigap is the type of insurance that attempts to fill the "gap" in coverage of services not covered by traditional Medicare.

387. **c.** Delayed gastric emptying

   The decrease in the rate of gastric emptying then slows the movement of oral medications into the intestine where the majority of medications are absorbed. Clearly, this is an issue for medications that are highly dependent on intestinal absorption.

388. **d.** 50 and 100 mL

   In older adults postvoid residual volumes between 50 and 100 mL are considered normal.

389. **c.** Benign paroxysmal positional vertigo

   The only diagnosis present that is consistent with these symptoms, is benign paroxysmal positional vertigo.

390. **c.** Alendronate (Fosamax)

   Ulcers in both the mouth and esophageal tract are possible side effects of Alendronate (Fosamax).

391. **b.** Following the organization's policies and procedures to generate high-quality care

   Nurse managers do not typically provide direct patient care. Instead, they are responsible for ensuring that the nurses on the unit are best able to provide high-quality care with the resources available.

392. **b.** Knowledge shared with patient, anticipated patient needs, and customized care

393. **c.** Metabolic syndrome

   Metabolic syndrome is a group of medical problems, that includes obesity and elevated glucose and elevated cholesterol levels. The presence of these risk factors substantially increases the risk of

394. a. Physical

Physical harm is the result of physical abuse.

395. a. Can be caused by bladder muscle weakness

Loss of muscle tone, loss of pelvic muscle strength, and bladder muscle weakness are all causes of incontinence in older adults.

396. c. End-of-life care often provides an opportunity to help patients complete important psychological and developmental tasks of aging

After assessing psychological and social issues, nurses consult with psychologists/counselors who can help older adults complete psychological and developmental tasks of aging.

397. b. Male gender, obesity, older than 65 years

Men have almost twice the sleep apnea rate as women, and sleep apnea occurs more significantly in adults over 50, especially in those who are obese.

398. c. High fiber in diet, increase fluid intake, exercise routines

Increasing fiber intake, increasing movement, and increasing fluid intake can all help alleviate constipation. For older adults, it is important that the increase in fiber go together with the increase in oral fluid intake to prevent the possibility of bowel obstruction.

399. b. Rule out delirium and depression as contributors to altered cognitive function

It is important to realize that cognitive loss is not considered normal. New onset of cognitive dysfunction should be evaluated, and depression, infection, and delirium should be ruled out.

400. c. 1,000,000

The estimated incidence of elder abuse is roughly 2 million per year. Hence, the correct answer is "c", exceeds 1 million.

401. b. Deep vein thrombosis

Immobility can lead to pooling of blood, increasing the risk of forming a blood clot. This, combined with a prothrombotic condition, will substantially increase the risk of a deep vein thrombosis (a blood clot in the leg).

402. d. Cataract

For patients experiencing cataracts, the vision is affected by a cloud-like haze covering the lens of the eye. This can make objects seem fuzzy, even at close range.

403. **a.** Polypharmacy

The risk of adverse drug reactions increases with the number of medications given. Polypharmacy, or the use of a high number of concurrent medications increases risk.

404. **d.** Respiratory

Posture can affect the ability of the pulmonary tissue to fully expand. Individuals who are severely kyphotic (hunched over) may have more limited tidal volume.

405. **d.** Osteoporosis

Hyperthyroidism is associated with osteoporosis. Similarly, a patient who is overmedicated with levothyroxine can also develop thinning of the bones. For this reason, all patients should have regular monitoring of their thyroid hormone levels.

406. **d.** Folstein Mini-Mental State Examination

The Mini-Mental State Examination is a standardized evaluation of cognitive status. The Barthel index of activities of daily living is a measurement of functional status. The Braden Scale measures pressure ulcer risk. The PULSES profile is a disability rating scale.

407. **a.** Ombudsman

The Ombudsman is charged with investigating complaints and attempting to find resolutions.

408. **c.** Decreased metabolic clearance of cortisol

As people age their metabolic clearance of cortisol decreases.

409. **c.** Active neglect

Active neglect is defined as the intentional withholding of care.

410. **d.** Pain

While all of these are symptoms that a patient may experience at the end of life, pain is the only physical symptom. The remainder of the answer choices are psychological symptoms.

411. **b.** Egg albumin

Some vaccines may contain egg albumin, a common food allergen. Patients with allergies to egg albumin can elect egg-free alternatives.

412. **c.** Actinic keratosis

An actinic keratosis is a rough, scaly patch on the skin that develops from years of exposure to the sun. It's most commonly found on the

413. **c.** Perform a needs survey of the staff to determine what they want to gain regarding leadership skills

    A needs assessment will help the presenter determine what the needs of the nurses on the unit are. The presenter can therefore make the experience more valuable by tailoring the presentation to the needs identified by the nurses.

414. **b.** Identifying specific self-care deficits

    The goal of a functional assessment is to identify specific self-care deficits.

415. **c.** Metformin (Glucophage)

    Chronic kidney disease (CKD) is common in older adults who are prescribed metformin (Glucophage) for type 2 diabetes. The U.S. Food and Drug Administration cautions that people with kidney disease should not take the drug because it could increase their risk for a potentially serious condition called lactic acidosis. This happens when lactic acid builds up in the bloodstream after oxygen levels in the body are depleted, raising concern for potentially inappropriate medication use. Medication safety deserves greater consideration among elderly patients due to the widespread prevalence of CKD.

416. **b.** Decreased liver function

    Older adults are affected by several physiologic changes that can affect drug metabolism. Among these are decreased excretion and decreased liver function.

417. **c.** Changes in the vaginal flora

    Changes in the vaginal flora can disrupt the natural balance of bacteria in the vaginal canal and lead to an increased risk of bacterial vaginosis (BV).

418. **c.** Urinary frequency, urgency, and nocturia

    These are signs of urinary incontinence. The other answer responses are indicative of other urinary problems, including UTI. The presence of a UTI should be ruled out prior to making the diagnosis of urinary incontinence.

419. **b.** 70 to 75 mm Hg

    There is a rule of thumb called the 70–70 rule suggesting that a normal PaO_2 for a 70-year-old is roughly 70. These values will be higher for younger adults and lower for older adults. Note that this is for arterial blood gas values. Normal oxygen saturation levels for older adults remain 95% or higher.

420. a. 24-hour recall

An excellent place to begin a nutritional assessment for both a younger and older adult is a 24-hour dietary recall.

421. a. Is reversible

The main distinction between delirium versus other types of cognitive problems in older adults is that delirium is reversible.

422. a. Power

If authority is not liked with power, a manager may be unable to successfully implement change.

423. b. Diminished visual acuity and glare

Common visual changes of cataracts include diminished visual acuity and glare. Other visual changes, such as diplopia, are suggestive of other visual problems.

424. c. Gingivitis

Gingivitis is an inflammation of the gums due to the presence of bacteria. Stomatitis refers to inflammation of the mouth and gums. Aphthous ulcers are commonly referred to as cold sores. Achalasia is a problem with the esophagus, which causes difficulty with peristalsis.

425. c. Intermittent claudication

Intermittent claudication is the name of a condition that causes cramping and discomfort in the lower extremities during exertion. It is associated with the presence of atherosclerosis, which limits blood supply to the affected area.

426. b. Psychological

Psychological abuse entails inflicting mental pain, anguish, or distress on an elder person through verbal or nonverbal acts; for example, humiliating, intimidating, or threatening them.

427. b. Memory loss, mood changes, weight loss

In the severe (late) stage of Alzheimer's, mental function (including increasing memory loss and significant changes in personality and behavior) continues to decline and the disease has a growing impact on movement and physical capabilities and is associated with weight loss.

428. b. Spiritual

Spiritual care is essential to improving quality palliative care. Studies have indicated the strong desire of patients with a serious illness and end-of-life concerns to have spirituality included in their care.

429. a. Confusion, tremors, weakness, diaphoresis

Confusion, tremors, weakness, and diaphoresis are all significant symptoms of hypoglycemia.

430. a. Either performance or capacity

Consistency in measurement is most important to achieve an accurate assessment of ability.

431. a. "A functional assessment is used to evaluate the overall ability of older adults to independently complete their activities of daily living."

432. d. Hip

Complications associated with hip fracture in older adults, reported by the CDC, include the following. A large proportion of fall deaths are due to complications following a hip fracture (one out of five hip-fracture patients will die within a year of the injury). Treatment typically includes surgery and hospitalization, usually for about 1 week, and is frequently followed by admission to a nursing home and extensive rehabilitation. One in three adults who lived independently before their hip fracture will remain in a nursing home for at least a year after the injury.

433. a. Brenner and Wrubel

Benner and Wrubel are known for their work on caring in nursing. Martha Rogers is known for her theory of unitary human beings. Madeleine Leininger is known for her transcultural nursing theory. Hildegard Peplau is known for her theory of interpersonal relations.

434. b. Amitriptyline (Elavil)

For patients in chronic pain due to postherpetic neuralgia, amitriptyline (Elavil) can help manage symptoms. Amitriptyline works both by reducing the depression, which can accompany chronic pain, as well as by blocking sodium channels.

435. c. Legumes and dried fruit

Legumes (beans) and dried fruits are excellent sources of iron.

436. a. Spirituality may provide a framework within which older adults search for meaning and purpose in life

Spirituality can be a critical aspect of end-of-life care, even for patients who are not religious.

437. c. A gradual decline of sensory perception

Gradual changes in sensory perception are common with aging. Among the most common are changes in vision and hearing.

438. d. Reed-Sternberg cells

Reed-Sternberg cells are characteristic of Hodgkin's lymphoma. They are large polynucleated cells, which are sometimes described as having an "owl-like" appearance. The Philadelphia chromosome is a genetic mutation associated with chronic myelogenous leukemia (CML).

439. d. Irritable bowel disease

Irritable bowel disease is often the diagnosis after other pathologies have been excluded.

440. b. Underdosing

The most common medication error for older adults is failing to take prescribed medication. Therefore, the problem is with underdosing.

441. a. Integumentary system changes

These are all normal changes of the integumentary system. There are actually decreases in elastin and subcutaneous fat that account for the thinness and reduced elasticity.

442. a. Insufficient CO_2 removal

An inability to exhale effectively will create problems with CO_2 retention. Therefore the answer is a. Insufficient CO_2 removal.

443. c. Confusion

A small percentage (about 5%) of older adults can have increased confusion and agitation when taking digoxin. The risk of confusion increases with the dosage.

444. a. Diminished central vision (scotoma), distorted images

The characteristic symptom of macular degeneration is the loss of central vision, and visual distortion.

445. b. Constipation

Constipation is a common side effect of opiate narcotics, which can be exacerbated in older adults

446. c. *Escherichia coli*

As in younger women, the most common infectious agent is *E. coli*.

447. **a.** Cataracts and macular degeneration

Both cataracts and macular degeneration can be managed by an ophthalmologist. In addition, glaucoma would also be managed by an ophthalmologist. Other disorders, such as vertigo and risk of falling, can be addressed by other members of the care team. Cerumen, ear wax, can be removed by either a nurse or by a patient at home using an over-the-counter preparation.

448. **b.** Motivating staff, empowering others to lead, and creating a vision

These three skills show leadership, as opposed to task-oriented behavior. While management of critical tasks is necessary, it is not a demonstration of leadership skill.

449. **b.** 1960 to 1970

Both Medicare and Medicaid were established in the mid-1960s.

450. **d.** Nurses should practice to the fullest extent of their education and training

The IOM report had four key findings:
1. Nurses should practice to the full extent of their education and training.
2. Nurses should achieve higher levels of education and training through an improved education system that promotes seamless academic progression.
3. Nurses should be full partners, with physicians and other health professionals, in redesigning health care in the United States.
4. Effective workforce planning and policy making require better data collection and an improved information infrastructure (IOM, 2010).

451. **a.** Continue a daily walking routine

Encouraging continued engagement with physical activity underscores the main principle of activity theory.

452. **b.** Poor glycemic control

An A1C of 8.5 is elevated. The American Diabetes Association recommends a target A1C for diabetic patients of 7%. Interventions should be recommended to lower the A1C level.

453. **a.** Anesthetic medication

Of these, anesthetic medication is the most likely to cause delirium.

454. a. Ask the patient to rate the pain on a pain scale

The best way to assess pain in a cognitively intact patient is to use standardized assessment tools. It is important to recognize the patient's self-report is the best indicator of pain. Nurses should not substitute their own judgment about how bad they believe a patient's pain is, or ought to be.

455. d. Both a and b

Weight loss and impaired wound healing are signs of poor nutrition in older adults. In malnutrition, serum albumin would be decreased, not increased.

456. a. Hydromorphone and diphenhydramine

A number of medications or combinations of medications can trigger delirium in older adults, including opioid pain medications (hydromorphone) and antihistamines with anticholinergic and sedative effects (diphenhydramine).

457. c. Veracity

Veracity is the ethical principle of truth telling.

458. a. It is legal and ethical to give a medication to treat symptoms at the end of life, even if giving that medication may hasten death.

Giving a medication when the intent is to treat a symptom is both legal and ethical, even if it hastens death. Giving medications with the intent to hasten death alone is termed euthanasia, and is illegal in most states.

459. a. Use a slightly lower tone of voice, repeat information as necessary

Because presbycusis is an inability to hear high-frequency sounds, it can often be accommodated by lowering the pitch of the voice.

460. c. Tardive dyskinesia

The concern with many first-generation antipsychotic medications is tardive dyskinesia, which refers to uncontrollable body movements.

461. d. All of the above

Excellent teaching would include not one, but all of these teaching techniques.

462. d. All of the above

Alzheimer's disease is more common in people with a genetic predisposition, those with Down syndrome, as well as those who are older than age 80. For patients with Down syndrome, the onset of Alzheimer's can occur quite young.

463. **a.** Allowing a resident to choose what to eat for lunch

Allowing a patient freedom of decision making demonstrates that the nurse values the autonomy of the patient.

464. **a.** Weight loss can help improve symptoms of osteoarthritis

Weight loss can substantially improve the symptoms of osteoarthritis, and may help patients delay joint replacement for many years.

465. **a.** TIA symptoms resolve more quickly

TIA symptoms resolve much more quickly than those of a CVA, typically within an hour, but sometimes within minutes.

466. **a.** Autonomy

Allowing a patient to have freedom of personal decision making demonstrates a commitment to autonomy.

467. **d.** Confidentiality

HIPAA provides for patient privacy and confidentiality. It restricts who can access and disseminate medical information about a patient.

468. **d.** All of the above

Lactose intolerance will restrict the intake of milk, a valuable source of vitamin D. Lack of sun exposure both from not going outdoors, and from covering up while being outdoors further decreases exposure to vitamin D.

469. **b.** Increase the level of feeding assistance provided

Often patients with Alzheimer's disease will lose weight in long-term care facilities because they may not receive the necessary amount of assistance at mealtime. Before making modifications to a patient's diet, it is necessary to assess whether the patient is receiving adequate assistance.

470. **b.** Decreased lubrication of the vaginal mucosa

Changes in estrogen levels affect the lubrication of the vaginal mucosa. This problem can be corrected with water-based lubricants or topical estrogen preparations.

471. **c.** The most common side effect is gastrointestinal disturbance

Cholinesterase inhibitors, the medications most commonly used to treat Alzheimer's disease, carry a high risk of gastrointestinal side effects.

472. **a.** "Would it be okay for me to ask you some questions about your sexual health?"

Assessment of sexuality often follows the PLISST model. This stands for Permission, Limited information, Specific suggestions and Therapy. The first step in the model is to ask permission from the patient to determine if they are interested in discussing sensitive topics.

473. **d.** The patient had a stroke caused by a thrombus

The patient could not have had a hemorrhagic stroke, as treatment with a blood thinner would be inappropriate. The use of warfarin indicates that the stroke must have been caused by a thrombus.

474. **a.** Bed alarms

Restraints can take many forms. A restraint is defined as any material or equipment that prevents free movement or access to one's body. Bed alarms allow free movement, and are therefore not characterized as restraints.

475. **b.** When the kidneys are not functioning properly, drugs tend to remain in the bloodstream longer, increasing the risk of toxicity

As people age, kidney function slowly declines. The kidneys of an 85-year-old person excrete drugs half as efficiently as those of a 35-year-old person.

476. **b.** A decrease in bladder muscle tone

With age there are increases in residual volume, decreases in bladder capacity, and decreased perception of urge. These factors, combined with a decrease in bladder tone, increase the risk of incontinence.

477. **d.** Both a and b

While most Americans would prefer to die at home, less than 25% actually do die at home.

478. **d.** All of the above

Normal aging-related changes affecting the respiratory system can all contribute to an increased risk for pneumonia in older adults.

479. **c.** Decreased tissue thickness

Skin becomes thinner with age due to loss of elastin, thinning of the epidermis, thinning blood vessel walls, and loss of fat below the skin

480. **a.** Decreased rate of peristalsis

In older adults the number of neurons in the human gut is reduced by about half of that found in younger people. Therefore, in up to 75% of

481. c. Chronic inflammation of the joints

All of the answer choices listed correspond to normal changes of the aging musculoskeletal system, with the exception of chronic inflammation of the joints. Joint inflammation is not a normal change of aging.

482. d. Bone reabsorption causing the bone to lose calcium causing decreased ability to produce material for the bone matrix

Changes in bone mineralization are the primary cause of changes to the skeletal system of older adults.

483. c. Confused older adults are more at risk for physical restraints than older adults who are not confused

Confusion can substantially increase the risk that a patient will be restrained.

484. c. A consequence of hypovolemia

In this situation the hematocrit is substantially elevated. An elevated hematocrit in an older adult is often a sign of dehydration—a hypovolemic state. The other answer choices listed would correspond to a low hematocrit.

485. a. "Do you have difficulty sleeping?"

This is the best example of an open-ended question. It invites the patient to provide more information about his or her sleeping patterns without judgment, and allows for further assessment of the patient's sleeping difficulties.

486. b. It is both legal and ethical to administer pain medication to a dying patient, even if the final dose of pain medication results in his or her death.

Nurses are permitted to administer medications for the purpose of symptom palliation. As long as the intention is symptom management, the action is legal and ethical.

487. d. To ensure the physical safety of the patient or other patients

One of the only valid uses of physical restraints is to ensure the safety of the patient or other patients. Once this immediate danger is no longer present, the restraints need to be removed.

488. b. Physical restraints

There are many effective interventions to reduce fall risk, some of which are listed as alternative answer responses. Physical restraints do not reduce fall risk, and they can, in fact, increase risk of fall injury in older adults.

489. **b.** Spinach

Of the foods listed, only spinach is high in vitamin K.

490. **d.** Poor staffing

While poor staffing can increase pressure ulcer risk, it is not one of the factors listed on the Braden Scale.

491. **d.** All of the above

Research studies have demonstrated that nurse staffing levels can have a profound impact on patient outcomes. For older adults, poor staffing levels increase rates of pressure ulcers and antipsychotic use. In addition, poor nurse staffing levels are associated with increased patient mortality.

492. **c.** Obesity

A modifiable risk factor is one that is under a patient's control. In this case, obesity is the only answer choice that can be changed, or modified, by a patient.

493. **a.** People with a weakened immune system

Because the shingles vaccine contains a weakened live virus, patients with a weakened immune system, such as those undergoing chemotherapeutic treatments or those with HIV, should not receive the vaccine.

494. **b.** Functional incontinence

Functional incontinence refers problems that prevent a person from getting to the bathroom on time. These can include changes in the musculoskeletal system.

495. **d.** Respiratory acidosis

A person with advanced pulmonary disease is unable to expel carbon dioxide efficiently. Because carbon dioxide acts in the body as an acid, this results in a net acidic state. Because that net acidic state is caused by a respiratory problem, it is deemed respiratory acidosis.

496. **a.** Older women may experience an absence of older male partners

Due to differential longevity, there can be a lack of partners for older women.

497. **b.** Contact the prescriber

A patient in severe pain requires immediate relief from pain. Asking the patient to wait until the next scheduled dose is not appropriate. The correct nursing action is to contact the prescriber so that additional pain medications can be ordered. Nonpharmacologic can be used as well, but are most effective for mild to moderate pain.

498. **b.** Administer the MS even though you know that it may hasten death

Under no circumstances should Narcan be used. It would cause the patient to have very severe pain. The nurse should administer the medication with the intent of relieving symptoms.

499. **d.** Contact the prescriber for an order for morphine sulfate SL

MS Contin cannot be crushed. Nurses should avoid placing IV lines in terminally ill patients. Therefore, the correct action is to contact the prescriber in order to change the medication to a route that the patient can tolerate.

500. **b.** Antiepileptics

Antiepileptic medications are effective treatment for patients with neuropathic pain, such as diabetics. In this group of patients, they can provide pain control, which is superior to that of opioids and NSAIDs.

Index

Printed in the United States